TESTING KNOWLEDGE

Before you start to read this book, take this moment to think about making a donation to punctum books, an independent non-profit press

@ https://punctumbooks.com/support

If you're reading the e-book, you can click on the image below to go directly to our donations site. Any amount, no matter the size, is appreciated and will help us to keep our ship of fools afloat. Contributions from dedicated readers will also help us to keep our commons open and to cultivate new work that can't find a welcoming port elsewhere. Our adventure is not possible without your support.

Vive la Open Access.

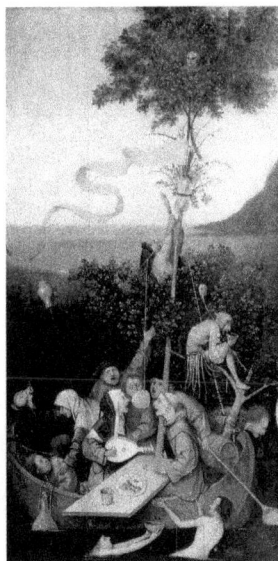

Fig. 1. Hieronymus Bosch, *Ship of Fools* (1490–1500)

First published in 2012 (*The Dingdingdong Manifesto*) and 2015 (*Testing Knowledge*) by Éditions Dingdingdong.

ding ding dong

Institut de coproduction de savoir sur la maladie de Huntington

English translation by Damien Bright published in 2021 by 3Ecologies Books/Immediations, an imprint of punctum books.
https://punctumbooks.com

This translation was kindly supported by the Fondation Universitaire de Belgique.

ISBN-13: 978-1-953035-45-5 (print)
ISBN-13: 978-1-953035-46-2 (ePDF)

DOI: 10.21983/P3.0307.1.00

LCCN: 2021935070
Library of Congress Cataloging Data is available from the Library of Congress

Book design: Vincent W.J. van Gerven Oei

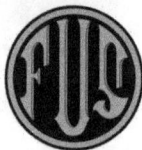

p. punctumbooks

spontaneous acts of scholarly combustion

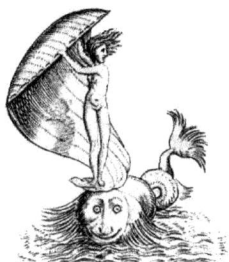

HIC SVNT MONSTRA

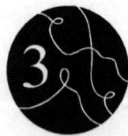

Katrin
Solhdju

**Testing
Knowledge**
Toward an
Ecology of
Diagnosis

Preceded by
**The Dingdingdong
Manifesto**
by Alice Rivières

Contents

Contents

Foreword

Alice Wexler

The call from my sister Nancy Wexler still resounds in my mind. "We found a marker!" she shouted over the phone. It was the summer of 1983 and Nancy had helped lead the team of geneticists and neurologists who had just mapped the gene for Huntington's disease (HD), an incurable hereditary motor, cognitive, and psychiatric disorder. Huntington's had claimed the lives of our mother, uncles, grandfather, and cousins over multiple generations. The discovery of the genetic marker – a variable stretch of DNA on chromosome four, located close to the Huntington's gene – was a giant step toward finding this gene and, we believed, developing a cure, or at least ways to prevent or mitigate the disease's cruelest effects.

The marker also made possible a predictive or presymptomatic test. Geneticists and neurologists had long dreamed of such a test and so too had many families like mine. Huntington's is an autosomal dominant disorder – meaning that each offspring of a parent who develops symptoms has a 50% risk of inheriting the disease. Typically these symptoms emerge in a person's thirties or forties, or even later, after children are born. A predictive test using the genetic marker – and ultimately the gene, discovered in 1993 – could indicate who among the offspring was free of the disease and who had inherited the abnormal gene and could pass it on to their children.

Many of us believed such a test, chosen freely by the individual concerned, could alleviate anxiety and dread in the lucky ones and at least facilitate future planning for the others. After all, a positive predictive test result – sometimes called a positive genetic diagnosis – did not mean you were ill in the present; it was strictly a prophesy for the future.

But what kind of prophesy? Predictive genetic testing turned out to be more complex, more challenging, and more ambiguous in its impact than we imagined, as Katrin Solhdju shows in her compelling and powerful book *Testing Knowledge: Toward an Ecology of Diagnosis*. As disclosed to Alice Rivières, a brilliant young French psychologist and writer, the predictive genetic test result for HD foreclosed any future other than deterioration and decline. "The doctors I met with were both terrified and fascinated by what they were having me do," writes Rivières. In possession of a powerful new technology, "a destiny-making machine," they suffered from a devastating failure of imagination that reduced "the multiplicities of tomorrow into a narrow, monolithic, flat, diagnosed sick future that stops the mind from the business not of grieving but of creativity."

Testing Knowledge builds on Alice Rivières's "ruinous" experience, which Solhdju interprets as both a cautionary tale and a provocation. She does not condemn a particular clinician or the (French) medical establishment for conveying a genetic test result in a brutal manner, as if it were a foreordained sentence to suffering. Instead she takes Alice Rivières's encounter as a starting point for improvisation. She asks how we can "cultivate an ecology of diagnosis that could place all actors involved in situations where they become capable of acting to the fullest extent possible." How can we develop narratives of Huntington's that fully acknowledge the variability of this illness, that situate those living with HD as actors rather than as passive victims, and that allow doctors and scientists to say "I don't know" in the face of uncertainty and ambiguity. She asks for "celebration without denunciation," that is, for celebrating hard-won biomedical advances – as of 2021, medications for chorea and clinical trials for gene-lowering therapies – while valuing alternative non-medical ways of knowing and responding to disease.

Even as they recognize the severity of Huntington's, Solhdju and Rivières reject the tragedy narrative and eugenic assumptions that run through much of the discourse on this illness. They ask instead, how can we live better with such a disease? How can we use Huntington's as "an opportunity to push thinking further?" As predictive and prenatal genetic testing becomes possible for a widening range of conditions, Katrin Solhdju shows us that, more than ever, we need the voices and knowledge of the users. We need our collective imaginations, fantasies, and "speculative narrations," from outside medicine and science as well as from within, to invent a future in which all of us, with Huntington's as well as without, may flourish.

– Alice Wexler, Santa Monica, California, January 2021

The Dingdingdong Manifesto

Alice Rivières

The Dingdingdong Manifesto

Don't look at what you're losing, look on what you've gained.
— My mother

In the beginning, when the world was just fifty centimeters long, there was Jeanne's inquiring face. A five-year-old face, flush up against the months-old fragment I then was, my opaque little mole eyes fumbling across this earliest of landscapes, my sister's face watching me. She smiles, I smile. I smile, she smiles. She gives me a quick slap, I cry, she smiles, I smile, she gives me another quick slap, I cry, she smiles, I smile. Late at night, we bond. My father bursts in, he sees me in my crib, he sees Jeanne as she leans over me and gives me a quick slap, he sees me cry, he slaps her, she cries, I cry, we cry, he gets angry. He doesn't understand. Jealousy, hostility, who knows what he assumes, but he thinks: here's a problem that needs fixing, separate them.

In the beginning and evermore, the limits of the Earth, its firmament, its floor, and its ceiling, they're Violette, who tackles everything with an eight-year head start, in other words an entire lifetime. Violette has a whole life on me, she goes on ahead, far in front, as big as the sky. She scatters her protective pheromones around me, something quakes in her when it quakes in me, our connection draws on resonance, and whether she's here or not, it's a thing of taut threads and stiff winds that carry fast and far. Early on, thanks to her, I learn that unconditional love does exist. At the same time, thanks to her, I learn that all love is not equal and that rarely is love so verily unconditional. I can act out, I can be away for years on end, I can fling myself every which way: she'll check if I'm still alive, sometimes gently reproach how I am mistreating myself, and then lets me go, loving me as always, which is to say without the slightest qualification, unequivocally.

There you have it. Nuzzled against me, one builds my self-awareness, and the other, awareness of the world around me, danger/no danger. (For a long time I thought none of this was mutual. I thought that for them we were just three sisters, and that I was the only one who saw it differently: the three-of-us.) My existence is stitched in double lining. And if I've forever sought to break these seams, to pierce them, to blaze my way through them, it's because wherever I go, they will always keep me together. When we learned that our mother had Huntington's disease, I hurried. I'm like that, I hurry, I rush things, I tear along, I rough draft, because all of my trials and errors are padded by my sisters, my double lining. It's not about rebelling or getting defensive about overprotective care, just the opposite: my sisters exist and so doing protect me, and so I am blessed with an incredible gift, the power-cum-duty to take risks. When my test results for Huntington's went red, they both jumped. When I'd rush into things, it often made them skittish, but this time they really jumped. I saw tremble with fear, body and soul, and my self-centered understanding of things finally came around to the fact that the three-of-us share a highly sensitive reciprocity mechanism: my sisters' lives also depend on mine. As we made our way in life through our respective bouts of trial and error, I had not concerned myself with this existential reciprocity, but ever since we learned that it was yes for me, no for Violette, and maybe yes maybe no for Jeanne, the world has really begun to shake: the problem is not that I'm struck, rather that the three-of-us are. Anything can happen to me on my own, indeed must happen to me on my own, because that way nothing happens that the three-of-us cannot deal with. But if something does happen to the three-of-us, there's a real danger it will all irreversibly unravel. That's why now I'm going to start at the end. It doesn't matter how the three-of-us came to be. It doesn't matter for now how many millions of minutes make up this singular thing, the three-of-us. The only thing that matters now is the emergency of dealing with what Huntington's has threatened to pollute in one fell swoop.

We were stunned, when Violette's test results came back negative three months after mine, by how devastated we both were, right when we expected we'd be jumping for joy. Violette's results were a good thing and they vindicated my conviction, steadfast from the very outset: Violette is to be spared from this bullshit. Violette, my compass, my very big sister, my little mother, founder of her very own clan that has since also become mine given how the three-of-us constantly entangle ourselves: spared from this bullshit, one and all. At almost that same moment, however, I was enveloped in a sphere of pure loneliness, a white and silent nucleus, that abrupt and radical removal from the world. (Maybe, when someone drowns, there's a point where they encounter this same loneliness, and at that moment they know that nothing is more real, more true – the slightest idea, the slightest concept is annihilated by the absolute purity of this loneliness.) I did not expect I would react by developing such an injury, such an open wound. With one blow, more than ever before, Huntington's had polluted me. It was not my test results but Violette's that led me to understand what was really going on, only then did the three-of-our pollution become clear: no for her, yes for me, and a tragic yes or an equally tragic no for Jeanne regardless. Hence what

I'm now fixing to imagine, a reaction in phase with the three-of-us. It's like the word game we so loved when we were kids, where you aren't allowed to give a yes/no answer. It's not the path of resistance, but of imagination. A merely defiant response will not overcome Huntington's pollution of the three-of-us. If we managed to invent the three-of-us, we can find something better than a yes/no answer for Huntintgon's.

Huntington's. The three-of-us learned that our mother had it first, which was difficult because she didn't know that we knew. Many years ago, when her father told her he was sick, he gave her an article on the subject from a medical journal, she tucked herself in a corner and read it alone, didn't tell anyone anything, and then ended up going for the blood test. Huntington's is an autosomal dominant disease, which means that if one of your parents is affected you've got a fifty-fifty chance of contracting it too, making you an "at-risk" person for the medical system. Since the genetic mutation was identified in 1993, to date it is one of the only predictive tests for a fully penetrant neurodegenerative disease. Technically, nothing could be simpler: you just take a blood test to find out if you have the bad version of the gene or not. Philosophically, ethically, psychologically, existentially, nothing could be more difficult, for Huntington's is a fully penetrant monogenetic condition: knowing you carry the abnormal gene means knowing with absolute certainty that one day you will develop the disease, yet not knowing whether that will be in three, five, ten, fifteen, or, if you're lucky, twenty years. My mother had the blood test done and then waited two years to go get the results. That was ten years ago, she learned she had the abnormal gene, then the disease, the very same condition that was incapacitating her own father, and throughout all this she did not tell a soul, especially not us. For ten years she did not say a thing. It's incredibly difficult to fathom: my mother's loneliness, my mother dealing with it all on her own, all this time. I cannot imagine it. And when I try to anyway, I'm overcome with tears of compassion: my thoughts stop and my head fills with terrible anguish for her instead. Much later, when we asked her why she kept it from us that whole time, she answered that she simply wanted to protect us. "Telling you such a thing when you were barely twenty years old, you must be mad! Why would I do such a thing?" She wanted to spare our twenties. To tell us or not to tell us: it was an impossible dilemma for her, and so we had to guess instead. And, after seeing her decline mentally and physically over so many years, without understanding what was happening to her, that's just what we did.

When the truth eventually came out, when we learned that Huntington's ran in the family and that our mother was sick, I already had a bit of an idea what to expect because of my training in psychology. I had hated that train-wreck of a class:

multiplesclerosisalzheimersparkinsonshuntingtons

Truth be told, it was more of a course on disability than anything else. Neurodegenerative diseases lead to the following physical disabilities and mental disorders, blah blah blah, there's nothing you can do about it, in fact nobody can do anything about it, so the best thing that you, future caregivers, can do is work with the disabled patient through mourning her normality. She's descending further and further into abnormality, but she doesn't know it, so you've got to help her recognize what's happening, in other words what she no longer has, or maybe she knows but won't accept it, and then you've got to help her mourn this loss. I had to write up all of this in my notes, and then recite it all on exam day to get a passing grade. I remember coming up with an exorcism ritual to cleanse myself of this foul nonsense straight afterwards. The classes taught us to transform people into anybodies (*quiconque*).[1] It wasn't a course in psychology but a course in anybodification (*quiconquisation*), and at that time I already found it infuriating. Yet two years later, when I crossed over to the other side, when I myself became a subject of medical anybodification, it did not matter that I was angry, it did not matter that I had worked "in the field" and had already given considerable thought to the matter – on certain medical practices' knack for capturing and purging, for instance. None of this protected me from the medical machine's remarkable power to anybodify me. Not one bit.

When we find out about her disease, all of a sudden my sisters and I have to revisit the last fifteen years of our mother's life, the last fifteen years of our own lives, the last fifteen years of our relationship with her. With this news, much of her odd behavior can be understood very differently. At the same time we are flung up against our own futures, now instantly and forever changed: Huntington's runs in the family, and each of us might have it, a fifty-fucking-fifty chance. At the time, the three-of-us are often overcome by waves of turmoil, by fits of anger, but rarely in unison. One of us whips into a rage, another slips into a Zen-like calm, the third falls somewhere in between, and the roles change from one moment to the next. That's still how it is for my sisters and me, we each dance a solo, taking turns, and we very rarely perform as a trio. One goes off and explores the hostile extremes while the others stay back and guard the base. When I learn of my mother's disease, I talk a lot, get tired, every day I think my understanding is getting better, stronger, deeper, but sometimes I trip and fall flat on my face, from really high up, and then all the meaning, all the meaning

---

1   Tobie Nathan, "En psychothérapie: maladies, patients, sujets, clients ou usagers?" paper presented at *La psychothérapie à l'épreuve de ses usagers*, Centre Devereux, Paris, France, October 12, 2006. Available online at http://www.ethnopsychiatrie.net/tobieusagers.htm.

built up all that time is flushed down the drain. Sometimes all that work makes my stomach weak, like I have indigestion. I get a little quieter than usual, I get stuck on repeat: I don't know, I don't understand. I forget how to start the thought process up again.

At this point, we don't talk about it with our parents. Our father is undergoing cancer treatment and our mother doesn't yet know that we're aware of what she's been going through. And we don't know how to go about telling her. My eldest sister and I go to see a therapist at a neurology clinic specializing in Huntington's hoping to better inform ourselves and get some advice on how to act towards our mother: how do we tell her that we know? Is she aware of her symptoms? What should we do to not upset her? The psychologist, who has never met our mother, her white lab coat doing all the talking, tells us that our mother is mad anyway and doesn't realize what's happening to her. "No matter how you go about things with her, it won't make a difference because she's anosognosic." This sinister word pollutes any attempt at defining Huntington's. It means that the patient is unaware of the horrific psychiatric and physical symptoms caused by the disease. The psychologist tells us our mother is anosognosic and she does it with a smile that drips with the magnanimous sputum of closure: what I'm about to tell you is how it is, *and it's for your own good,* you'll have to get used to it. Regarding our own peril, she suggests we think of a coin: it's just a matter of heads or tails. We leave her office more dazed than ever. I find somewhere to hole up, far away. I need to be alone. I don't do anything except bury myself in Rachmaninoff, in his language of war. For two weeks I turn myself inside and out, and end up deciding to get tested. All in all, I'd spent six weeks thinking about it. First I wanted to get tested, then I didn't, and in the end I decided I wanted to know. We weren't designed to know our destiny before it happens, says one expert. I agree, but when you have got the option to know *anyway,*

you automatically become a bit different as a human being. I wanted to know so as to not be sick. To rid myself
of medicine and disease. I was convinced I was not a carrier, I wasn't shouting it from the rooftops, but I was both
terrified and confident: I don't have this thing. If I had it,
I'd have felt it, I would feel it. Feel what, exactly, I didn't
rightly know. But I also knew that if I didn't get tested, I
would be wracked with doubt, like a house haunted by a
troublesome poltergeist that wreaks havoc day and night.

Jeanne is less frightened than Violette and me at this
time, she didn't go with us to see that hospital therapist,
she isn't corrupted, her connection to it all is much simpler and more candid, and so one fine day, without any
warning whatsoever, she turns to our mother, uncorks
a bottle of champagne (because for us champagne and
announcements go hand in hand) and tells her we know
that she is sick. She brings her up to speed and everyone
cries, not so much of sadness as of tenderness: we have
found each other again, after all these years of senseless
separation, we are together once more. My mother is immediately overwhelmed with relief at no longer having
to live alone this knowledge, because she blamed herself
terribly for not saying anything yet would have blamed
herself even more had she told us, for it would inevitably have poisoned our lives – our lives, that which she
holds most dear. Our mother's reaction is the exact opposite of what the specialist therapist had predicted. She
is entirely aware of what is happening to her, she is not
the slightest bit mad and can understand everything we
tell her as long as we communicate things clearly. This is
one of the first lessons we learn: to see someone as anosognosic – as the psychologist had encouraged we look
on our mother – sows confusion, misunderstanding, and
estrangement (we're normal, they're abnormal). It places
this person in a world that isn't quite ours anymore, the
very world of anosognosia. The belief that Huntington's
and anosognosia go hand in hand, and the associated im-

pact on how you behave towards those affected, causes as much anosognosia as the condition itself. I therefore came to regard anosognosia with the greatest suspicion.

I set off on the path to genetic testing. I am told it will take time: three months, maybe more. First I meet with a neurogeneticist, who explains that I have to see a psychiatrist, a psychologist, a social worker, and then another geneticist before getting the blood test done. I manage to get around the social worker and the psychiatrist. I meet with a psychologist who asks me why I have decided to get tested. I explain everything candidly, and her response is that I appear quite unemotional, that I should let my feelings out. What about a slap in the face, how's that for feeling? Or maybe she would rather watch me and my emotions yank the drawers from her desk and roll around on the floor, sniveling and in tears? The other geneticist is an old man who scrawls impenetrable diagrams full of arrows on bits of paper while he talks. I leave with his scribblings, more confused than ever about what they are all going on about. Meanwhile, I google Huntington's disease six ways from Sunday and become more and more terrified at what I find. Soon enough, I stop being able to type the words "Huntington's disease" into Google's search bar without literally starting to shake. My investigations grind to a halt. I have to go back and see the first neurogeneticist again, to let her know whether I've decided to go ahead with the blood test or not. It feels like a driving test: I have to prove who I am, they have to think I'm strong enough to quell their fears that I'll kill myself because of them, yet I also have to appear upset enough not to come across as emotionally shut down. It's a tricky line to walk, but I end up pulling it off and they allow me to get my results two months after the start of the testing process, the hallmark of a successful applicant. They draw two vials of blood, because the results have to be double-checked by two different labs.

In the weeks leading up to the test results, the more
the night draws on, the less tired I become. Lying in bed,
my mind wanders, eyes wide open in the darkness, and
I go looking for this hypothetical foreign body that, un-
beknownst to me, might have been living within me this
whole time. Huntington's disease. I don't find or feel anything in particular except for the sheer terror of the expedition itself. Often I have strange bodily sensations, I
experience astonishing ways of thinking and feeling, tin-
gling, electric shocks, dissociations, murderous thoughts,
a lot of desire. My thoughts jump seamlessly from one
subject to the next, or the exact opposite occurs, they
come to a complete standstill, like the ceiling above me.
I experience all of these things, yet remain aware enough
throughout to know that for the most part these phenomena stem from that same question – "have I got this
thing in me?" – and were they not always there, making
my body their home sweet home. That very question sets
off this rollicking jig of physical sensations and sudden,
strange thought processes, not so much moments of
weakness as moments of panic in which my brain works
at lightning speed to find an answer. Soon enough I'm
barely sleeping or eating, all I can do is think, and I don't
want to do anything else. Hours go by like seconds while
I investigate the possibility of this occult marriage, Huntington's and I. I now know that the question of whether
or not I was a genetic carrier was not alive. In the words
of William James, the hypothesis that I could be a genetic
carrier was a dead hypothesis because it did not appeal
to me "as a real possibility."[2] The question was a zombie

2   "Let us give the name of hypothesis to anything that may be pro-
     posed to our belief; and just as the electricians speak of live and dead
     wires, let us speak of any hypothesis as either live or dead. A live
     hypothesis is one which appeals as a real possibility to him to whom
     it is proposed. If I ask you to believe in the Mahdi, the notion makes
     no electric connection with your nature, it refuses to scintillate with
     any credibility at all. As an hypothesis it is completely dead. To an

question, and I was its prey. It produced no vitality what-soever, and was maybe even dead itself, but when this question captured me as it did, I was wholly and utterly at its command. With the test results a few days away, having looked long and hard and finding nothing much at all other than the side effects of the question itself, I latched onto the certainty that I was not sick.

On the day itself, I went to see the neurogeneticist for a third time. Emmanuelle came along with me. She had been by my side every step of the way, playing my girlfriend at each appointment (given they asked me to play a part, why not take it all the way and pretend to be homosexual?). Another close friend also came along, and it is fortunate they were there because I have no recol-lection whatsoever of the moment when my test results were revealed. My memory refused to capture it and my two friends now carry the memory of this instant for me. I can only remember the neurologist telling me it was bad news, and that she herself was surprised because, she said, more often than not in her experience she did not need test results to recognize, know, or sense that some-one had the disease. And that she hadn't "seen" any such signs in me. She delivers the sentence as my CAG number: 44.[3] No need for a second opinion. The number is well above the threshold that separates those who carry the disease from those who do not. She then turns to Em-manuelle and tells her how dreadful it will be for family and friends, and that she needs to quickly start getting

Arab, however (even if he be not one of the Mahdi's followers), the hypothesis is among the mind's possibilities: it is alive. This shows that deadness and liveness in an hypothesis are not intrinsic prop-erties, but relations to the individual thinker." William James, *The Will to Believe and Other Essays in Popular Philosophy* (New York: Dover Publications, 1956), 2ff.

3   CAG stands for Cytosine-Adenine-Guanine. More than thirty-six repetitions of this glutamine on the fourth chromosome indicate the presence of the gene responsible for Huntington's disease.

help herself. Not content with cursing me, she dunks my friends in her pox as well. All I can think about is fleeing this place as quickly as I can, but first I have to pretend to listen to her advice about coming back to see them and getting counseling from their team of therapists. I make a silent oath never to see her again. I close my ears and manage not to break down. (My emotions and feelings are chunks of intimacy that she does not deserve.) Outside in the corridor, five minutes later, I collapse for a moment. I wait until I've left the hospital to scream.

Throughout this entire journey, I never felt as if anything other than a predetermined set of reactions and behavior was expected of me: "good behavior," the kind that would or would not grant me what I wanted: to take the test. Taking the test – because from the moment it existed, from the very moment it had been created, I had to take it. The simple fact that the test existed made it utterly irresistible to me. When I learned of my mother's disease, all my bearings past and future skipped town and the test revealed itself to me, radiant with the glory of its absolute certainty. Because there was a test, I could not do without it when erecting even the slightest of solid foundations for my future. Every hypothetical construction of self I would devise independently of the test was necessarily based on hope, on a "maybe not," one step removed from the denial of reality that we psychology practitioners so gleefully condemn.

To devise such an instrument, the predictive test for Huntington's disease, such a resolutely vertiginous instrument, and then to allow it to become the withering process I underwent, is, I believe, not only a deep disappointment but the sign of a very grave, unforgivable failure of medicine. The test is a destiny-making machine. Going through with it means witnessing the radical and immediate transformation of your inner truth, that constantly quivering kaleidoscope, into the simple truth of a medical definition. My kaleidoscope and medical definition do not share the same mode of existence. I am willing to incorporate a medical definition into my kaleidoscope, but a medical definition is not able to integrate my kaleidoscope without destroying it down to the last shard. In the case of Huntington's, the test had transformed medicine into the provider of singular forms of truth, truth-which-cannot-lie, the specificity of which is to crush all others. As the testing process wore on, the geneticist kept saying that if the outcome were bad, what she'd have to tell me would not be a diagnosis (of my current state) but information (about my future state). Yet when it comes to a genetic condition like Huntington's, where the genetic anomaly is fully penetrant, the distinction between information and diagnosis is far too subtle to be of any use. The test is formidable. I do not regret having taken it, because there's no point regretting the inevitable. However, I do regret that it was invented. Had it not been invented, I would not have taken it, and I would have had to construct something else from the news that my mother had the disease. I realize today that I had two possible destinies: not "with or without Huntington's," but rather, "with or without the test."

Experts carefully argue that testing is not so much a matter of diagnosing as "revealing genetic status." Sure, why not! But in that case why stop there? They should work with us on this new riddle (*énigme*) of theirs: what does it mean for a person to have their genetic status revealed? There's nothing trivial about a revelation, it's a big deal, and I agree with geneticists when they talk about revelation to describe the predictive test. But I do not agree with the conclusions they draw from such an experience. Revelation does not inform you. Quite the contrary: it transforms you. It can either make you sick or make you better: it all depends on what you do with it. As for me, and I know I'm not alone, the test stopped being a curse the moment I actively separated and protected myself from medicine.

I blame the scientists and doctors for making an offer that was too good to resist for someone in my position,[4] and then displaying such galling incompetence, not so much towards me as towards their own creation, the test. The process itself reflects this problem every step of the way. The doctors I met with were both terrified and fascinated by what they had me do. And from this strange vantage point, the best they could offer me was depressing and corrosive stereotyping. The only pronouncements they made were condemnations: your mother is insane, your life is a coin toss, a matter of heads or tails, it's going to be dreadful for friends and family, there's no treatment, you are very healthy for now but when you get worse you will come and work on your disability with us, what's that, you plan on adopting a child?! ... (expression of horror/sympathy). Thinking through Huntington's disease together, thinking through this terribly enigmatic business, was never an option for them. Perhaps they aren't there for that because they are doctors and not philosophers. Perhaps they are just there to treat you and make you better. The problem with Huntington's, however, is that there is no making you better. The disease has no cure.

What do I blame them for? Not that they can't do anything to help (they're not omnipotent, I realize that), rather, that they opt for a default professional viewpoint bereft of humility, and cowardly to boot. If you don't have the technical means to make me better, yet you have got a hold of this test – an instrument too powerful for you to handle – try and take the opportunity to learn something, try and push yourselves a little: the situation is

4 Early thirties, single, and without children. The decision to get tested or not is intrinsically linked to your personality, age, relationship status, and whether or not you have children, in which case the curse inevitably takes hold of their futures. Thankfully, these days a vast majority of at-risk people decides not to undergo the testing process.

not business as usual so don't act as usual. Don't look at me all, "been there, done that." You're telling me my future is Huntington's and then you say I'm not emotional enough? Do you realize what an absurd and destructive position that is? The problem is not Huntington's incurability; the problem is that the test holds you as you hold it. It demands that you be able to make something living out of it. But you wouldn't dare. You are cowards, your conscience is sitting pretty while we struggle through testing, and you take every opportunity to belittle us as we go.

Therein lies my anger. Those who get tested give you a chance to raise your standards, and you do not take it up; quite the opposite, you want to anybodify us as usual. And so doing, not only do you not fix us, you make matters worse. You make our situation even more depressing than it already is, because you block off possible escape routes and flatten our futures. You concoct a Huntingtonian future for us that is bland, mediocre, handicapped, insane, predictable – a definition wrought by you alone – without thinking for one second that it might be possible to have Huntington's and completely eschew the model you've created, to be doggedly out of step with your definition. It never occurs to you that you do not own us, that we could be something other than your creatures. And how could you? Your power to transform humans into medically conforming creatures, into beings defined from head to toe by you alone, this power is such that, once caught within its cogs, it becomes incredibly difficult if not impossible to disentangle and defend oneself. Most of the time, getting sick is a double bind: disease on the one hand, medicine on the other. Should a sick person begin to challenge her treatment, she soon finds herself in pain and alone. At best, her aggressive behavior is explained away to her as the result of feeling that, as a sick person, she is the victim of some sort of injustice for which her anger can find no other outlet. At worst, say if she's a smoker and happens to enjoy a drink from time to time, she is told that what is happening to her is her fault anyway. How dare we question those with the power to make us better? A power relationship such as this, which quashes and silences any semblance of a challenge, is profoundly unhealthy. I'm lucky: medicine cannot do anything to help me, which is why I'm free to criticize it.

My indignation is greater still when it comes to psychology's attitude toward Huntington's disease. If medicine considers that thought production is none of its business, so much the pity. For psychology to take a similar view is, however, astounding. As always, in the testing process for Huntington's disease, psychology intervenes when medicine hits a dead end. And when the moment comes for psychology to take up this glorious and ambitious charge, to generate healing in spite of it all, it too sets to work on its default setting, bathing me in preconceived and pitifully inadequate notions like "the grieving process." Psychology too is determined to treat me like it's been there and done that, and so doing serves medicine's needs and not my own, applying its tools to reinforce the impact of the medical curse. To encourage me to work on mourning my normality is not only stupid but also dangerous. I'm not dead yet. Maybe I shouldn't have been born, but I'm not dead yet.[5] And like most of us, I was never normal. Telling me to grieve for my normality places me within a normative program of long-term, existential withdrawal that destroys all the singular possibilities contained within my experience of becoming-Huntington's before they've even been explored.

I understand medicine's difficulty as guardian of the genetic test, whether it likes it or not. The art of the test is

5   These days, women who carry the disease or the genetic expansion and who decide to conduct a prenatal test when pregnant, are advised to have an abortion if the results indicate the fetus is also a genetic carrier. Carrying the disease means being forced to live alongside this eugenic logic.

in its hands, and yet medicine is ambivalent about making it available to the infamous "at-risk" population, particularly after having observed a rise in suicide attempts from individuals who test "positive" for the disease.[6] And if there's one thing medicine hates, it is killing people. Indeed, its sole obsession is making sure that people do not die, or if they do, that it is absolutely not medicine's fault. Medicine is right to fear suicide attempts from individuals who follow through with the predictive testing process. This risk is embedded within the test's very outcome. My hypothesis is that, as things currently stand and in terms of their respective effects, the disease and the test are one and the same. Testing deforms your life, whether you carry the disease or not. If it shows that you are not a carrier, you have nonetheless been possessed by the prospect such that you are irrevocably transformed. Upon learning the good news, what do you make of this stunted metamorphosis? Not to mention the rift that such a result creates with those in your family who are sick. How do you rejoice without placing an irreparable distance between you and them, without feeling guilty? If the test says you are a carrier, your path in life takes a degenerative, downhill turn. Checkmate. The process can fuss over you all it likes, with its social workers, psychiatrists, and psychologists. It does nothing else but confirm and empower the withering malediction uttered by the test. Under such conditions, depression and suicide attempts are hardly unexpected. In fact, I'm surprised anyone survives the experience at all.

Through this powerful labeling process, where the only vanishing point provided by medicine is a generalized withdrawal – deterioration – it immediately oc-

6   Elisabeth W. Almqvist et al., "A Worldwide Assessment of the Frequency of Suicide, Suicide Attempts, or Psychiatric Hospitalization after Predictive Testing for Huntington's Disease," *The American Journal of Human Genetics* 64, no. 5 (May 1999): 1293–304.

curred to me that suicide was the only alternative with enough power, counterpoint, and emancipatory freedom. The thought seized me straight away: if I'm going to deteriorate, I may as well finish it right now. I'm not interested in that future, I reject it and if, as it seems, I'm not able to reject it, if the only thing I'm offered is to help me accept it, then I'll stop all this right now because I'm not interested in accepting such a thing. I refuse to consider that life is deterioration. I have never, for instance, considered that aging is an unrelenting phase of decline, that it is set to be that equation they drum into us: the older you get, the less you get. Less strength, less health, fewer memories, less sexuality, less flavor, less knowledge. I've never got my head around that kind of thinking and if, after all that, because of Huntington's, I'm forced to think of myself as someone who will never again be moving forward, then too bad, I'll end it now one way or another. I began to think this way from the moment I was polluted by the medical definition of Huntington's and, more generally, by the medical definition of my genetic status. From this pollution onward, committing suicide was therefore the only sensible answer to an absolutely senseless medical proposition.

I managed to rid myself of this pollution by quarantining away medicine, by realizing that what ails me is not so much Huntington's disease as a disease for which medicine has found a definition but can do preciously little else. By understanding that medicine defines nothing, that you have to take its definition for what it is: a stop sign, beyond-this-point-we-are-no-longer-competent, in other words, an object still needing to be thought through and defined. By understanding this, I began to breathe again. Medicine takes its own limitations as a working definition. The test makes Huntington's disease into something phantom-like: an entity holly and yet possessive and terrifying. Each time a patient takes the test and is told of her Huntingtonian future, one of these disturbing creatures enters the world. The testing process and its design principles of precaution and anybodification address this creature the only way they know how: domestication by way of notional deterioration. As such, the situation resembles a state of war. Medicine is my enemy for it insists on wanting to brand me with a moribund future. It can be my ally if and only if it agrees to fashion a surfeit of intelligence (i.e., vitality) from what's happening to me.

It took me four years to get better. Not from Huntington's disease, but from the psychological trauma I experienced when my test results were announced. I call them "tragic spells": they're just as powerful as magic spells but they make you rot, reducing the multiplicities of tomorrow into a narrow, monolithic, flat, *diagnosed sick* future that stops the mind not from grief but from creativity.

I recovered because I met a neurologist and HD specialist who agreed to work on an antidote with me. This doctor's patience and common sense are impervious to assault and her commitment and empathy are extraordinary. As I see it, however, these qualities are not what make her so effective. (I should say, I do not doubt that within the medical profession, of which I have been so vehemently critical here, there are many who possess these same qualities). I believe her ability to make this antidote stems from one thing only: her humility towards the disease, an a priori humility. She could have said no for the simple reason that it's not her job, which is to treat the truly sick and ignore pre-symptomatic carriers sickened by the test, like me. But she offered to do it, and most importantly, she offered knowing full well that neither she nor I had any idea what we were getting ourselves into. From the moment we were both of this mind, the antidote wasn't that hard to make. It consisted of a slow and gradual reinjection of everything that had been eroded by the test: doubt, uncertainty, hesitation, the maybes, what-ifs, and feel-your-ways. In other words, she put her stock in pragmatism (following what this experience could teach us) rather than determinism (knowing in advance what would happen). Along the way, within the very core of this abstract, bland, and empty place called the genetic-coding-of-Miss-A.R.-with-Huntington's-mutation, she knitted, strand by strand, the possibility of releasing surprise anew, and displacement, disorientation, zigzagging, depth, perspective, insight, unexpected knowledge – simply put, a dose of living-living.

In a few words, my task now is to invent a solution akin to an antidote in its nature and its action. To devote your entire being to devising a truly operational solution is an undoubtedly vitalizing path – so much so that I often wonder if life and the endeavor to create this solution are not one and the same. When it comes to developing this solution, anything that cannot be put to the test or into the world is of no interest. In this sense, my process is one of pragmatist research, drawing on the Jamesian notion of a wager.[7] For William James, when you're faced with a painful, stultifying, and moribund existential conundrum, it's time to have a wager, a somewhat therapeutic wager with a revitalizing thrust. James points out that once I've designed this wager, I have to set about building up everything that will help me pull it off. It's like he's asking me not just to bet on a horse, but also and above all, to make sure the horse wins, by taking care of it, readying it, by riding it and, who knows, why not, even by becoming the winning creature myself.

Intelligence is the relationship that thought forges with reality, the world, and adjacent sources of intelligence. Intelligence cannot exist, cannot unleash itself, unless it is extended through contact, in an interactive mode. To emerge and develop, it must enter into an almost loving relationship with whomever and whatever

7   See the truly therapeutic writings of William James, especially *The Will to Believe*.

it encounters. Here I wish to suggest that the conditions that would ensure my solution are grounded not in the energies of despairing loneliness but in collective emulation. Inventing an alternative understanding of Huntington's disease is an extraordinarily ambitious project needing robust means and a number of able minds to see it through. The greatest risk posed by such an experiment – having-Huntington's-disease – is that the sickness becomes separated from its own intelligence, which would kill both things: a patient's intelligence and the potential for intelligence inherent in the disease itself. My wager is that Huntington's disease provides an opportunity to push thinking further.

Dingdingdong was born to give me the means to win this wager. Dingdingdong is a collective whose sole vocation is to create a living and operational way of thinking through Huntington's. This collective does not intend to collate general information about the disease, or raise funds to treat those affected by it, which existing organizations do a remarkably good job of already.[8] It's not a federation but a gathering of individuals driven by a common, vital concern for creating innovative thinking from their experience with the disease. The collective's communication strategy could be termed *proffercation*: no condemnation without a counterproposal. It's not a collective *against* anything – against the disease, for instance – but rather *for* building something that does not as yet exist, above all, a specifically Huntingtonian way of thinking whose current lack exacerbates the suffering of those affected by the disease.

Dingdingdong is first the call of three bells whose voices ring true and clear and yet, like the three-of-us,

---

8 For France, see *Huntington France,* http://huntington.fr/; *Huntington Avenir,* http://www.huntingtonavenir.net; as well as Huntington's message boards such as *Huntington-Inforum,* http://www.hunting-ton-inforum.fr.

are linked together, an echo of folly ringing in their hearts. It's a warbling call, high and loud, to cut through the brouhaha of routine thoughts and warn of an urgent need to slow down. It's a call that chimes with Huntington's, so much so that for the three-of-us it became an acoustic compact: say Dingdingdong when you're too scared of Huntington's, and say Dingdingdong when you want to laugh or scare off Huntington's.

How do you think when thinking deteriorates?

How do you think through how to think when thinking deteriorates?

How do you think through how to think when thinking deteriorates while thinking is deteriorating?

How to write about how to think when thinking deteriorates?

How to write about how to think when thinking deteriorates while thinking is deteriorating?

My circumstances naturally lend themselves to the idea of founding a collective. I have an urgent need to strengthen the three-of-us. I have an urgent need to have an army of my own, to protect the three-of-us from all contamination. Given that one day the disease will limit the means and faculties I currently enjoy, I want to put safeguards in place now, so that these limitations will be balanced out by other intelligences that can continue to provide adequate nourishment for my soul, despite – indeed, by way of – these same limitations. Such safeguards are not meant to guard us from madness, but to keep madness safe in its intrinsic state, to encourage its expression, so that it might be released and inform the world with its fragile teachings. Today, I can be this safeguard for others but one day I will surely need others to take my place.

This project means I must consider myself to be Huntingtonian. However, all I can say at this stage, given where my thinking is currently, is that I do not yet know if I am Huntingtonian. Not because I am yet to display any symptoms of the disease, but because it all depends on how the collective tackles this sprawling entity, the constellation called Huntington's. Unlike many diseases, especially mental ones, the identification of a gene specific to Huntington's disease (IT15 on the 4th chromosome) should close off the question, "am I Huntingtonian or not?" There is no doubt that my own gene bears Huntington's mark: my CAG repetitions exceed normal levels. I'm at 44 on this scale-that-does-not-lie – over 36 and you've got Huntington's. My mother has 42, like her father. My elder sister has 17. The existence of such a "reliable witness" – abnormal CAG repetitions – makes this question obsolete when in fact it is open, open and fascinating for a majority of diseases, for which no reliable genetic markers have yet been found.

Schizophrenia is a good example. One of the collectives concerned by this disease does not believe in calling itself a gathering of schizophrenics because, in light of its members' own experiences, it feels that the term "schizophrenic" is less pertinent than "voice hearers."[9] The members of this collective hear voices, it's complicated, it's uncomfortable, and at times painful, it may not be normal, but that doesn't make them schizophrenics (particularly because "schizophrenic" immediately seems to mean one thing only: the imperative to take antipsychotics for the rest of your life – which is something some choose not to do, in any case, *not at all costs*). They prefer, and I agree with them on this, to call themselves "voice hearers" because this designates that they have an ability that other "normals" do not, and further, that the goal of their treatment is not to eradicate this additional ability but to live a better life with it. Their question is not, "how do I treat my schizophrenia?" but rather, "how do I live a better life with my voice-hearing ability?"

9   See *Hearing Voices Network,* http://www.hearing-voices.org.

Thanks to the voice hearers, I can rephrase my question. The problem is not: to be or not to be Huntingtonian, but rather: what do I gain from defining myself as Huntingtonian? It's about transforming a tragic question into a Jamesian question: what is the better wager? What is the wager that conjures the most vitality? What do I win and what do I lose by suggesting I am Huntingtonian? The stance taken by some Autistic people is helpful for thinking this question through. Unlike the voice hearers, some Autistic people not only accept but uphold their Autistic status, yet only insofar as adopting such a position means acknowledging the singularity of their world, a world which is theirs and resolutely not ours: Autistic culture. They therefore do not locate themselves in a hierarchy that runs from normal to pathological, but rather in the simple acknowledgment of difference. In other words, these individuals with Autism rally behind the medical syndrome known as Autism, yet they do so in order to arrive somewhere far beyond obedient adherence to its medical definition (handicap, deficiency, other-than-normal). This Autistic culture movement leads, for instance, to the discovery of another culture, diametrically opposed and foreign to theirs, neurotypical culture, which is to say normal people's culture, which they cheerfully conceive of as some kind of incurable pathology.[10] The fact such groups exist is an extraordinary boon to me. If I'm at all confident in my efforts, it's because their audacity is infectious.

(I won't hide that founding a collective is somewhat entangled with my own personal writing project, as I also need the collective to continue this work. The project, titled Tahitidouche,[11] is a literary and existential project.

10 See, for instance, the "Institute for the Study of the Neurologically Typical" project, archived on http://web.archive.org/web/20101225092135/http://isnt.autistics.org/index.html.

11 Some of this project's ideas will be developed within the foam laboratory and research unit of Dingdingdong, the Institute for the Co-

It's the starting point for the search for my own language, for my own sense of reason and of madness. Writing is the most precious and reliable means at my disposal for hosting the creations to which my Huntingtonian life is now bound. Because writing is both how I remember and how I create. I am unable to create anything outside of writing and I am unable to remember anything that is not written down. If Huntington's disease is a world waiting to be discovered, she – Huntington's is indeed female, as in the French language the words "earth" (*monde*) and "disease" (*maladie*) are feminine – needs her own language, her own mythology, her own founding texts. I need the collective to inform the mode of writing which can speak, describe, and bring Huntington's into existence, thanks to the shared experiences it will provoke and thanks to the Huntingtonian us-jectivity (*nousjectivité*) it will reveal. I have no doubt whatsoever that the raw material of this us-jectivity will be text.)

Dingdingdong's challenge is to establish a system of knowledge production that articulates the collection of individual accounts with the development of new pragmatic proposals, with a view to helping its users (*usagers*)[12] – carriers, patients, kin, caregivers – to live with Huntington's honorably. Original forms of collaboration between users, researchers (medicine, philosophy, sociology, history), and artists (fine artists, writers, videographers, choreographers...) are needed for an endeavor such as this: probing this disease as unchartered territory and discovering narrative forms capable of relating this adventure as it unfolds.

In this sense, there is no one goal, no predetermined production to be achieved, but rather an expedition to be carried out, an expedition whose trajectory cannot be

production of Knowledge about Huntington's Disease. See https://dingdingdong.org/.

12 See this volume, 50n3.

known in advance. By ridding ourselves of a specific goal, we're delivered from that same panic felt by Huntington's carriers who have undergone the predictive test and who are continually shepherded toward the disease as the sole apex, endpoint, and inescapable destination in life. Yet everything changes if we refuse to be blithely captivated by this eerie attraction to the distant and dangerous planet pointed out to us by the medical profession. Far off, and far removed from our current condition, held aloft as some kind of solar system at the heart of which lays a fatal star, the sun of death. Everything changes if we choose, instead, to look at our feet, to look all around us, just behind us, or just in front us: if we begin to observe the ways in which we're already in contact with this thing. Everything changes if we consider what is happening right now. We're already making contact. In other words, it's already an event.

This planetary metaphor is no coincidence.[13] With considerable nuance, Lars Von Trier's film *Melancholia* relates the different possible ways of facing a foretold catastrophe. In brief: a planet called Melancholia is about to crash into Earth and we witness a family's last days – a couple, their sister in law, and young son. The husband character, played by Kiefer Sutherland, believes tooth and nail in the official/scientific assessment that the planet will just brush past Earth before continuing its onward trajectory. He is so deeply convinced that when he realizes the scientists were wrong or lied (we never really find out, and for once this isn't the point), he kills himself by swallowing the vial of poison his less trusting wife procured. Her character, Claire, played by Charlotte Gainsbourg, is, on the other hand, constantly afraid: we see her, now para-

---

13 I follow, on tippy-toes, in the footsteps of Émilie Hache, here, who deploys Lars Von Trier's *Dogville* to literally make the reader experience the moral positions of a societal controversy. Émilie Hache, *Ce à quoi nous tenons* (Paris: La Découverte, 2011).

lyzed with fear, now gesticulating wildly, possessed by terror and unable to do anything but submit to it, until the very end, when she gives in and entrusts herself, body and soul, to her sister Justine, played by Kirsten Dunst. Justine (whose impossible "human" matrimony we followed in the first half of the film), is the only person able to experience the planet's encounter. She shares this ability to not shy from reality with the property's horses, who make their own journey, as if to say: the ways that lead us to this encounter are varied and infinite, because they reveal our very inner natures.

Melancholia is as much the story of this encounter as it is of the disease, its necessary prelude: a strange affliction that befalls Justine, a nameless sickness, or rather a sickness that does not so much bear the name of the approaching planet, but a sickness that is itself the approaching planet. In other words: Justine is not melancholic. Melancholia has taken Justine. Under such circumstances, Justine suffers from not yet having encountered what she already belongs to. Like a fish out of water, Justine is sick from having to exist outside her natural environment, and her condition worsens until she encounters that which, at last, makes her become who she really is. This encounter gives rise to an amazing scene in which, bathing naked in its glow, Justine makes love with the planet. From this moment on, Justine regains her appetite and her strength. She is cured.

I believe you can compare the existential dissonance that afflicts Justine with the impossible encounter experienced by carriers of Huntington's disease – insofar as current medical knowledge sets the conditions for such an encounter, in any case.

It's worth remarking that, in this film, "official" science aspires to be reassuring and constantly intones that nothing bad is going to happen, unlike what happens with Huntington's disease. Yet, indeed, when it comes to the encounter itself the net effect is the same: "don't worry, nothing's happening" and "red alert, disaster imminent!" conjure a paralyzing fear. One is confronted with something for which no answers can be found, but of which one thing is certain: it's really happening. Dingdingdong is an encyclopedic endeavor whose object is not Huntington's disease but the encounter with a neurodegenerative genetic disease understood as a mysterious planet that has already taken some of us. The researchers involved in this collective – whether they are carriers, patients, doctors, philosophers, sociologists, artists, writers – are committed to using their know-how in order to experiment with ways of proudly coming to know an experience, something scouted out by its users yet which may concern us all: living with a genetically foretold disease.

Testing Knowledge:
Toward an Ecology of Diagnosis

Katrin Solhdju

›

Introduction

> *The truth of an idea is not a stagnant property inher-*
> *ent in it. Truth happens to an idea. It becomes true, is made*
> *true by events. Its verity is in fact an event, a process: the*
> *process namely of its verifying itself, its veri-fication.*
>   – William James[1]

Medical diagnoses transform those who receive them, dividing a person's life into a before and after. They dramatically reveal the implacable entanglement of the biological life of the organism with the biographical life of the subject. When danger befalls biological life, a person, along with her entire life story, comes undone. The trouble with diagnostic situations is that they force a translation upon factual and objective knowledge produced by scientific techniques, for instance regarding the genetic status of a living organism, turning it into an announcement made to *somebody*. They thereby acquire, so to speak, the "wild" or untamed power to transform a person in her entirety. If diagnostic enactment is capable of radically calling the existence of its addressees into

---

1   William James, *Pragmatism: A New Name for Some Old Ways of Thinking* (New York: Longmans, Green, and Co., 1916), 201.

question, then those involved, practitioners and patients alike, are in urgent need of tools and techniques for sharing the responsibility that invariably goes hand in hand with such power.

This is an especially challenging undertaking in diagnostic situations that force medicine to reckon with its own limitations. What happens when a test confirms that a person – or more accurately her blood, urine, skin, or limbs – has or will develop a disease, yet no corresponding treatment exists? Medical practice cannot then operate as curative art towards the conditions it diagnoses. This inability to act suggests therapeutic powerlessness, which produces profound disarray, if not breakdown, among doctors, patients, and loved ones alike. Those involved rarely admit this to one another, and so all too often a powerless doctor will confront an equally powerless patient with extremely upsetting information about her body, and hence her life today and to come, yet can provide no constructive propositions concerning what happens after diagnosis.

This kind of diagnosis is not simply *in*formative, it is *trans*formative. It transforms each and every actor involved, along with their broader relationships. Nonetheless, it can provide relief in some cases, for example, by finally putting a name to a set of painful symptoms after a long and hitherto fruitless search. Diagnosis then puts an end to an uncertainty that is often harder to bear than the certainty of suffering from a severe disease or, from a medical point of view, the desperate quest for the right diagnosis. However in other situations – and this is especially so for predictive tests, also known as presymptomatic tests, enabled by contemporary genetics – diagnosis, or the positive stipulation of a prognosed disease, risks becoming a sentence or, to be precise, a curse that overpowers not only a person's present and future but also, assuredly and *retroactively,* her past.

In such cases, medicine can indeed provide factual, scientific answers. It can say whether or not an abnormal mutation is present in such and such an organism and at such and such a location. However, practitioners are often bereft of adequate forms for communicating such diagnoses. They lack ways of speaking and of acting that might meet the complexity of the knowledge they possess and its attendant implications. This failing cannot be simply chalked up to the shortcomings of individual doctors, to a dearth of empathy, or to psychological misadventure. It arises in case after case and should instead, I submit, be regarded and interpreted as an effect of the epistemological drive inherent to modern medicine, a drive which some historical excursions can help clarify.

Diseases and Their Milieu

One of the conundrums of modern medicine is the way in which an entanglement of epistemological, ethical, moral, and legal features consistently separates facts, deemed scientifically objective, from values, deemed subjective and unmoored from these same facts. At first, this imperative drew strength from medicine's need to assert itself as a scientific discipline, much like physics, chemistry, or biology. The demands of patient autonomy and enlightened consent, which have been foundational categories of medical ethics and law since the 1960s, lent subsequent support. Admittedly, such concepts gave patients (their autonomy recognized at last) the ability to refuse treatment advice from doctors (their paternalism overcome, at least in theory). Autonomy so construed amounted to a reactive veto power. Yet this did not give patients the ability to intervene into the reality of the disease that befell them, as something with which they lived. Expert knowledge over this experience remained the privilege of doctors. As historian and philosopher of science Alfred Tauber observes:

Patient autonomy, rather than being corrosive of professional privilege, may actually reinforce physician authority; autonomy tends to be a negative right (in that a person has the right to refuse treatment) rather than a positive right (a person cannot generally demand a particular treatment). [...] Indeed, physicians have incorporated informed consent into their practice as a means of improving patient satisfaction, and perhaps most importantly, shifting responsibility to the patient provides a potent tactic to combat malpractice suits.[2]

Pertinent albeit disillusioned as this remark may be, other practices concerning a wide range of conditions have emerged in recent decades. These indicate that diseases can transform themselves, for doctors and those affected alike. Through know-how and practices that depart from science in the strict sense of the term, it is even possible to alter their so-called *natural history*. The existence of these conditions is undeniable and painful, and yet for those living with them what they really are is never determined once and for all. Instead, their existence is constantly subject to new experiences and new questioning. The truth(s) of these phenomena, it turns out, can take multiple forms and can vary in relation to the *milieu* in which they unfold. The Intervoice Network provides an instructive example. It is an international user initiative that assembles people to whom psychiatry has addressed a schizophrenia diagnosis.[3] In taking up the term

2   Alfred I. Tauber, *Patient Autonomy and the Ethics of Responsibility* (Cambridge: MIT Press, 2005), 60.

3   The Dingdingdong collective employs the term "users" to refer to all of those who participate in a culture of usages with Huntington's disease, whether because they are sick, at-risk, loved ones, caregivers, physicians, etc. See also Emilie Hermant and Valerie Pihet, *Le chemin des possibles: La maladie de Huntington* (Paris: Les Presses du réel, 2017).

"voice hearers,"[4] members of this movement do not simply reject schizophrenia as a diagnosis. They counter it with techniques for seeking constructive ways of living with the voices they hear. They have devised a peer-based training system, by and for hearers themselves, to better share and perfect these techniques. Their initial observation was that in most cases, only some and not all voices heard are unpleasant or threatening. Training therefore aims to provide those concerned with the know-how needed to cultivate, with discernment, their singular ability to hear voices that no one else can – rather than reduce them to silence through drastic pharmacological treatment, which tends to be minimally effective anyway. This network also provides training for psychiatrists, with a growing number choosing to participate. This is no small measure of the movement's success. By learning new techniques from users (in the sense of experts of a particular culture of usages), these doctors are hoping to enrich their own practice. In such light, voice hearers not only transform their own usage of illness but have also begun to substantively influence the *natural history* of schizophrenia, including the clinical course of the disease. They follow in the wake of other efforts, led for instance by Autistic or Deaf people, that also undertake user-oriented coproduction in order to intervene upon and transform the very reality of what ceases to be a disorder – an impairment to be suppressed at all cost – and instead becomes a *singularity*.

User groups nurture genuine *expertise*. French psychologist and writer Tobie Nathan demonstrates how these collective projects put medicine – and especially psychiatry[5] – to the test. These groups demonstrate that ways of

---

4 For an overview of this movement, see Angela Woods, "The Voice-hearer," *Journal of Mental Health* 22, no. 3 (2013): 263–70.

5 See, for instance, proceedings of the conference "La psychothérapie à l'épreuve de ses usagers," held in Paris October 12–13, 2006, available online at http://ethnopsychiatrie.net/textcolloq.htm.

living, co-existing, and making do with sickness – whether from a clinical or caregiving perspective or one set by those directly concerned – do more than transform its public perception. They have a profound effect on what I term, following Étienne Souriau and Bruno Latour, the *modes of existence* of disease.[6] At the same time, they orient, in deep and lasting ways, the rewriting of the *natural history* of disease. The reality of a particular sickness is only partially captured by medico-scientific disease categories; it is also a thing of lived experience, an illness unfolding for a given set of people, at a given time and within a given milieu. Indeed, we should consider these dimensions of lived experience alongside diagnostic procedures and frameworks, as constitutive elements of the milieu or *oikos* (household) of diagnosis. Put directly: an ecology of diagnosis must account for all of the elements that make up its milieu. For example, an "Autism" diagnosis *is not the same thing* when heeding the assumption that symptoms express a lack of maternal affection (the "refrigerator mother" theory), as it is when heeding calls from activist user communities to acknowledge their inherent singularity, which includes asserting the existence of a distinct Autism *culture*. An Autism "diagnosis" is henceforth transformed; it is no more the same than a pneumonia diagnosis before and after antibiotics, a diabetes diagnosis before and after insulin synthesis, or a multiple sclerosis diagnosis before and after the advent of pharmaceutical treatment that, although not a cure, affords considerable control over how the condition unfolds.

In such light, diagnosis is not simply a communication of knowledge from one person to another or from the laboratory to the consulting room, wherein that knowledge

6 Étienne Souriau, *The Different Modes of Existence* (Minneapolis: University of Minnesota Press, 2015) and Bruno Latour, *An Inquiry into Modes of Existence* (Cambridge: Harvard University Press, 2013).

remains inherently neutral despite its secondary subjective and psychological effects. Instead, diagnosis must be understood as a manifold (*complexe*) of facts/values made up of a condition's many layers of existence. To study these modes of existence, which is to say the milieu of a given diagnosis, is, therefore, critical for understanding how diagnostic practices that run the risk of becoming a veritable curse, overwhelming the creative capacities of those concerned, can, instead, become opportunities for coproduction, if not of assured vitality then at least of metamorphosed vitality in the face of the lived experience of disease.

Opening the Box

In order to become capable of foregoing a reaction of passive disarray in the face of devastating diagnoses that threaten to unleash a veritable pox, and to turn instead towards actively constructing new possibilities, it is necessary to open the Pandora's box of diagnosis as a situation.

Taking a historical and genealogical approach, I will first elucidate how contemporary diagnostic systems (*dispositifs*) came to be, the legacies that they bear, along with the disciplinary, epistemological, ethical, and legal ideals and regulations that they heed. This will provide the grounds for constructive criticism of these same features. In so doing, my aim is not so much to denounce medicine and its practitioners, but rather to heighten our sense of the different features through which diagnostic situations become so intense as to require a rethinking of the ways in which they distribute the capacity to act. Consider the mere existence of a range of literature from practitioners themselves, such as *The Difficult Conversa-*

tion, Breaking Bad News, and so forth.[7] These documents convey a pressing demand to make sense of the "how to" of diagnostic activity on the part of doctors themselves. While a sign of genuine good will, above all they reflect the need for an undertaking that operates at multiple registers and gathers together a diverse array of disciplinary skillsets, an undertaking that nurtures thinking together, fosters a multiplicity of knowledge and practices, and is able to produce less stereotypical and reductive *versions* of diseases and their diagnosis.[8] There are two preconditions for steadily building such an understanding. Firstly, that all actors involved (doctors, caregivers, patients, and loved ones) agree to share their respective disarray. Secondly, that we begin conceiving of practices that can not only "dissociate the symptom from the person"[9] but can also reconnect a person to the attachments and affiliations that make up her world in order to put a stop to the process in which she is severed from any consistent reality in the name of the laws of nature.

This book begins by tracing the genealogy of a most unusual diagnosis, the predictive test for Huntington's disease, to convey a sense of how its inherent violence is made manifest. The second chapter examines the extent to which such manifestations of violence adumbrate a history of modern medicine. I will attempt to recount this or rather these stories with a view to better understanding the characteristic failings of current diagnostic

7   Edlef Bucka-Lassen, *Das schwere Gespräch. Patientengerechte Vermittlung einschneidender Diagnosen* (Cologne: Deutscher Ärzte-Verlag, 2005); Christian Lüdcke and Peter Langkafel, *Breaking Bad News. Das Überbringen schlechter Nachrichten in der Medizin* (Heidelberg: Economica Verlag, 2008).

8   My use of the concept of "versions" draws on the work of Vinciane Despret. For a discussion of this term, see Vinciane Despret, *Our Emotional Makeup: Ethnopsychology and Selfhood* (New York: Other Press, 2004).

9   Tobie Nathan and Isabelle Stengers, *Doctors and Healers* (Oxford: Oxford University Press, 2018), 70.

practice and identifying the favorable conditions for replenishing this devastated framework. The task, therefore, is to elaborate a better understanding of the situations under consideration in order to *problematize* their attendant difficulties *otherwise* and thereby orient toward new possibilities for becoming with disease. The book's third and final chapter draws upon these stories to develop propositions adequate to a singular setting. This setting is characterized by a radical asymmetry between, on the one hand, forms of knowledge and power that can transform a person in her entirety and, on the other, a lack of therapeutic know-how. These propositions must, in practice and in effect, prove themselves capable of enriching the imagination of those exposed to these situations, regardless of their position, such that they thereby develop new capacities for action. They should add consistency to these diagnostic milieus; in other words, they must prove capable companions for the shared construction of a better "ecology of diagnosis."

1

The Many Lives of Testing

*My wager is that Huntington's disease provides
an opportunity to push thinking further.*
– Alice Rivières[1]

Following my encounter with Alice Rivières, and in learning of her experience with the genetic test for Huntington's disease, I felt the pressing need to work towards an ecological understanding of diagnosis. "We weren't designed to know our destiny before it happens [...] but when you have got the option to know *anyway,* you automatically become a bit different, as a human being,"[2] writes Rivières in the "Dingdingdong Manifesto." Some years ago, she "succumbed" to the force of attraction of predictive genetic testing. "The simple fact the test existed," she writes "made it utterly irresistible to me. [...] Because there was a test, I could not do without it when erecting even the slightest of solid foundations for my future."[3] The test promised, or at least appeared to promise, to help her know her future. Yielding to its seductive power, she decided to submit (or to subject herself) to the process of medical, psychological, psychiatric, and social

---

1   Alice Rivières, "The Dingdingdong Manifesto," this volume, 37.
2   Ibid., 23–24.
3   Ibid., 28.

evaluations that precedes the actual test, and then to undertake the genetic test itself.

Predictive testing for Huntington's disease (HD) takes on singular meaning because of the fact that, to this day, the disease remains incurable. Making sense of the many difficulties testing raises in such circumstances requires a definition of the condition itself. Yet this task raises a veritable avalanche of questions for a project like Dingdongdong, a collective project committed to thinking, inventing, and instantiating counteragents or antidotes to ostensibly hopeless representations of the disease. How do we *introduce* Huntington's disease when the stated purpose of our collective labor is to actively *transform* it through sophisticated forms of "knowledge coproduction"? Dingdingdong adopts a critical stance toward the reigning definitions, discourses, and practices of Huntington's disease, given that we aspire to iterate and institute interesting forms of contact and life *with* it. Under such circumstances, are we able to appeal to biomedical knowledge or to genetic and neurological explanations, and if so how? Conversely, if our task is to make novel and less hopeless *versions* of HD become true – which means making them truly real – had we better not, for now, reserve an answer to the question of what this sickness *verily* is?

I fear, however, that postponing definition in the name of precision would risk jeopardizing the perspicacity of Dingdingdong's enterprise, whose very force derives from drawing contrasts with established and official *versions* of HD. Yet it would be incorrect to assume we aim at challenging the accuracy of biomedical knowledge of the disease. Rather, we stand against the assumption that life *with* this particular condition, and with disease in general, can be wholly or largely distilled within scientific and medical knowledge thereof.

When it comes to diagnosis, Huntington's is something of an exception to the extent that it can be detected "predictively," in other words, before the onset of any symptoms. By way of a "simple" blood test, at-risk persons can receive a practically conclusive prediction of whether they will or will not experience the many symptoms of this "neurodegenerative" disorder.[4] In this same way, it is possible to determine whether such persons' children or grandchildren also carry a risk. For if a person does not carry the mutation, they cannot transmit it – the genetic legacy ends with them. This is because HD is autosomal dominant, monogenic, and shows complete penetrance. The first characteristic, in the rules of genetics, indicates that any person having one parent who is a carrier is at a 50/50 risk of inheriting the defective gene. The second means that the disease develops in the presence of a single modified gene. The third implies that any person carrying the relevant genetic mutation not only bears a higher than average risk of falling ill but that they will inevitably develop symptoms sooner or later – unless they happen to die of other causes beforehand.

The American physician George Huntington provided the hitherto most complete description of HD's nosology in 1872, and for quite some time the disease was known as Huntington's chorea. It is difficult to find comparisons for the condition in light of its symptomatology. This includes multiple motor, neural, and behavioral changes that manifest over the years, with unpredictable highs and lows. People typically present symptoms between

4   The first long-term studies subsequent to the test's uptake have shown that something of a "genetic gray area" exists, albeit a very slim one. See Nayana Lahiri, "The Genetic 'Gray Area' of Huntington's Disease: What Does It All Mean?" *HD Buzz,* April 22, 2011, http://en.hdbuzz.net/027, and Regine Kollek and Thomas Lemke, *Der medizinische Blick in die Zukunft. Gesellschaftliche Implikationen prädiktiver Gentests* (New York: Campus Verlag, 2008). In addition, "neurodegenerative" is placed in scare quotes because, after interviews with persons with the disease as well as their loved ones and caregivers, Dingdingdong holds that patients do not experience a strictly linear decline but rather a zigzagging progression.

the ages of thirty and fifty. Involuntary and sporadic muscular spasms termed chorea (from *choreia,* the Greek word for dance) along with psychological disturbances and various changes in personality tend to signal the insidious onset of a sickness that only death brings to halt. While psychoactive medication such as antipsychotics and speech and physical therapy offer partial relief for individual symptoms, to this day there is no cure nor stabilizing treatment.

Loss of balance, altered and impaired cognition, marked difficulties with vocal expression and agglutination, as well as various psychological challenges from depression to psychosis – this harrowing and extensive combination of symptoms mean that HD is often regarded as the "most horrible," the "most monstrous" and "the most cruel" of diseases. It was long known as "Saint Vitus's Dance" and thereby associated with a state of possession.

The hereditary nature of the disease helps to explain this tendency towards demonization, which medical practitioners have been known to relay. In point of fact, potential HD carriers – so-called "at-risk persons" – can observe among family members what they inevitably perceive to be heralds or omens of what, for them, is coming. Such is how most persons at risk of developing Huntington's disease live: well before undertaking their own diagnostic or therapeutic treatment, they already live with the sickness in various guises through one or more loved ones. They live with medicine's varying degree of powerlessness towards them. They regard themselves as witnesses of their own future, of their own suffering and death, well before they themselves fall ill. Huntington's disease *accompanies* entire families across generations and often leaves the impression – from within as well as without – that these families are truly cursed. This disease therefore plays a significant part in forging the identity of afflicted families, often taking the form of a taboo with sinister and insistent powers that incontrovertibly reveal themselves in the symptoms of parents and grandparents, brothers and sisters, aunts, uncles, and cousins. All too often, Huntington's disease is a well-kept family secret: it is unspeakable and must go untouched yet it relentlessly pushes its way to the surface and stakes a claim to the realm of the visible and the perceptible. It should now be apparent that the predictive diagnosis of HD runs the risk, because of what it is and what it does, of replicating an existing curse. For this very reason, it requires truly careful consideration.

A New Kind of Foreknowledge

Beyond the confines of the molecular biology laboratory where facts are made, genetic testing's technical simplicity meets with a correspondingly complex and troubling situation. The very possibility of knowing the future calls forth a cascade of questions, which have bearing for those directly concerned as well as the physicians, social workers, psychotherapists, ethicists, and other actors involved in some capacity with the process leading up to the test. One set of questions relates to conditions of access. Another concerns how to appropriately handle the announcement of a diagnosis, namely the moment in which laboratory information becomes subject to translation within the clinical relationship that binds patient to practitioner. HD's particular genetic and clinical configuration lends a heightened sensitivity to questions over the manifold possible and feared effects of such translation. Indeed, because of the radical ways in which HD brings ethics, morality, family, politics, and the law into question,[5] physicians and geneticists along with so-

5   Huntington's disease is one of the only late-onset diseases for which early detection is available, although this does not constitute a form of "screening," strictly speaking, given the ongoing lack of curative

ciologists, psychologists, bioethicists, and public health experts have long pointed and no doubt will continue to point to the condition as an exemplary case.

The exact identification of the gene responsible for Huntington's inaugurated the possibility of a *direct* genetic test for the monogenic disease in 1993, thanks to the work of an international consortium of scientists who located the gene on the fourth chromosome's short arm. They discovered that greater than thirty-six repeats of the CAG triplet that encodes the amino acid glutamine is an indication of the mutation's presence and thus HD's future expression at the level of the organism. As its name implies, an indirect genetic test came before the "direct" one. Preceding the latter by a decade, the former followed from the discovery of a marker "coupled with the Huntington's gene."[6] This allowed genetics to "determine the status of at-risk persons with a high degree of probability."[7] However, conducting this indirect form of predictive genetic testing required genetic material beyond that of the individual at-risk person querying their genetic status. Until the gene's precise location in 1993, this earlier form of linkage-testing was only possible when cross-generational analysis and comparison within the same family could establish whether a person inherited the allele acting as bearer of the genetic marker from one parent or another.

As such, the indirect genetic test was only practicable in a limited number of cases because its subject's family

treatment. The condition remains a source of significant social stigma; following their doctors' advice, persons who learn of their "positive" status adopt strategies of secrecy, if only to protect themselves and their families against the haunting administrative and financial consequences of disclosure.

6   Thomas Lemke, *Veranlagung und Verantwortung. Genetische Diagnostik zwischen Selbstbestimmung und Schicksal* (Bielefeld: Transcript Verlag, 2004), 31.

7   Ibid.

needed to be large enough to furnish the necessary genetic material. Hence, the task's complexity came to be
directly correlated with its effects upon and among the
families it came to involve. This prior form of testing accordingly highlights the critical function played by family in Huntington's disease, so much so that the condition
is often fundamental to the identity of those involved
– albeit negatively – and distinctively connects them
to the rest of their kin. It should come as no surprise,
therefore, that family also played a crucial role within
medicine in distinguishing HD from other diseases. At
the age of twenty-one George Huntington wrote "On
Chorea," an article distinguishing HD from other forms
of developmental and infectious chorea, referring to it
as "hereditary chorea." It was only possible for him to do
so, however, because he was in possession of reliable data
drawn from across multiple generations of sick people in
his town. In fact, both his grandfather Abel Huntington
and then his father George Lee Huntington had served as
the local doctor before him. It can be assumed that their
experiences fed into George's careful study and analysis
of the symptoms and modalities of transmission linked
to what was then known as "Saint Vitus's Dance" or simply "that disorder."[8] Because he was able to access medical histories that had been meticulously maintained for
the same families across multiple generations, the young
Huntington was in a position to articulate one of the central biological rules of heredity for the disease – unaware
that he was doing so at almost exactly the same time that
Mendel was undertaking his landmark study of heredity
on pea plants. The rule would come to be known as "the
dominant mode":

8   George Huntington, "On Chorea," *Journal of Neuropsychiatry and Clinical Neurosciences* 15, no. 1 (Winter 2003): 109–12.

But if by any chance these children go through life without it, the thread is broken and the grandchildren and great-grandchildren of the original shakers may rest assured that they are free from the disease.[9]

In 1872, Huntington worried that his description of hereditary chorea would not hold "any practical importance" for his colleagues and so offered it "merely as a medical curiosity, and as such it may have some interest."[10] A century later, however, the disease's heritability would play an essential role in genetic research.

At a 1972 conference held in Ohio to mark the centenary of George Huntington's article, psychiatrist Ramón Ávila-Girón showed a short black-and-white film that his colleague Americo Negrette had made in a small village situated on the banks of Venezuela's Lake Maracaibo, attesting to the high local incidence of HD. Attending this session was Nancy Wexler, a young psychologist from a family impacted by HD who would later play a decisive role in advancing genetic research on the disease. The film's content and dramatic imagery were striking and affecting, but so too was the fact that the high concentration of HD in this one area made for an almost natural laboratory in which to acquire the breadth of material needed to understand its functional mechanisms. Inspired by research using homozygotes (persons receiving a given gene from both parents[11]) to study family anemia resulting from inherited high cholesterol, Nancy Wexler and her colleagues launched a research project at Lake Maracaibo in 1979 in the hope of finding homozygote carriers of the HD gene with and through whom to advance

9   Ibid., 111.
10 Ibid., 112.
11 The history of genetic research is filled with homozygotes; they feature so heavily because of their precisely calculable risk for hereditary diseases.

scientific discovery.[12] Thanks to the meticulous collection of genetic and clinical material at the site, the extended group of researchers was able to identify the genetic marker for HD in the years that followed – the initial hypothesis, it turned out, was a generative one.[13]

It should be said, however, that although the new indirect test became available for use, it tended to produce inaccurate and even more frequently "uninformative" results – meaning that they were too inconclusive and therefore unreliable or uncertain to reveal to at-risk persons. Nancy Wexler, Michael Conneally, David Housman, and James Gusella, all members of the team that discovered the marker, insisted this was only the beginning. It was to be the beginning of a long journey towards the complete understanding of Huntington's disease, an understanding they manifestly hoped would play an important role in the fight against it. Looking back, Carlos Novas offers a penetrating analysis of the implications of this "journey":

The journey which they speak about involves the search for a potential treatment or cure, a journey which may hopefully not only alleviate the suffering caused by this disease, but also transform predictive genetic testing into a gateway for access to therapeutic regimes, and not, as it is at present, a complex technol-

12 The idea for the Venezuelan project came up in the context of the Congressional Commission for the Control of Huntington's and its Consequences, which Nancy Wexler continues to lead. She is also the president of the Huntington's Disease Foundation, established by her father Milton Wexler.

13 I am weaving this story from the extraordinary retelling provided by Alice Wexler, a historian and Nancy's sister. See Alice Wexler, *Mapping Fate: A Memoir of Family, Risk, and Genetic Research* (Berkeley: University of California Press, 1996). I would also like to warmly thank Alice for her precious comments on the manuscript, as well as for her generous foreword

ogy for the management of genetic fate by those who are at risk.[14]

Despite locating the gene for Huntington's disease in 1993, the journey was far from over. This was because the discovery itself did not bring about any preventative or therapeutic solutions.

The genetic research boom of the 1980s and 1990s gave new hope to geneticists, physicians, patients, and their loved ones. They hoped to take effective control of biologically predetermined fate, a fate whose unfolding could now be foretold. Yet these hopes remain largely unrealized to this day, in the case of Huntington's disease and many other quarries of the genetic sciences.[15] Genetic knowledge provided and provides but a rudimentary starting point for developing effective therapeutic practices. What's more, even in these early days there was hardly a scientific consensus on wishful thinking. Consider how, as early as in 1992, Nancy Wexler describes the dramatic consequences of the asymmetry between genetic knowledge and its inability to produce clinical advances:

> The natural trajectory of human genome research is toward the identification of genes, genes that control normal biological functions and genes that create genetic disease or interact with other genes to precipitate hereditary disorders. Genes are being localized far more rapidly than treatments are being developed for the afflictions they cause, and the human genome project will accelerate this trend. The acquisition of

14 Carlos Novas, *Governing "Risky" Genes: Predictive Genetics, Counselling Expertise, and the Care of the Self* (Boston Spa: British Library Document Supply Centre, 2003), 200.

15 Even though today more and more promising fundamental-research projects as well as clinical trials, experimenting on the possibilities of gene-therapy, are on their way.

genetic knowledge is, in short, outpacing the accumu-
lation of therapeutic power – a condition that poses
special difficulties for genetic knowing.[16]

To be sure, the detection of disease continues to achieve
greater breadth, speed, and accuracy. Yet in most cases
such knowledge hardly ever comes with power, whether
preventative or therapeutic, directly or indirectly. Wexler's penetrating insights draw attention to this asymmetry, which she considers foundational to genetics as a
field; with the completion of the Human Genome Project
in 2003, this asymmetry became dramatically obvious to
the public at large.

Regardless, it is no longer possible *to think* Huntington's disease outside of a world in which such forms of
knowledge are available and whose mere existence influences the sickness and those it touches. No sooner
was the gene located than everything changed. Thereafter, any and all at-risk persons have no choice but to
take a position when it comes to the possibility of prediction, even if they oppose the test and decide they do not
want to know. By making such a decision they become
a moral actor – whether they like it or not.[17] Hence, not
only does the test's mere existence refashion medicine's
relationship to HD. It also dis- and reorganizes practices
of knowledge sharing around risk that families had developed over generations. While often oblique, gestural,
and uncertain, such practices gave rise to careful ways of

16 Nancy Wexler, "Clairvoyance and Caution: Repercussions from the
Human Genome Project," in *The Code of Codes: Scientific and Social Is-
sues in the Human Genome Project*, eds. Daniel J. Kevles and Leroy E.
Hood (Cambridge: Harvard University Press, 1992), 211–43, at 218.
Emphasis mine.

17 The work of Lotte Huniche explores this question in depth. See, for
instance, her "Moral Landscapes and Everyday Life in Families with
Huntington's Disease: Aligning Ethnographic Description and Bioethics," *Social Science & Medicine* 72, no. 11 (2011): 1810–16.

experimenting with half-truths about one's status – and even outwitting it. In light of this test, important questions abound about the right to know and not to know and the anonymity of those involved.

In her book *Mapping Fate: A Memoir of Family, Risk, and Genetic Research,* published in 1996, Alice Wexler, historian and sister of Nancy, offers a simultaneously fascinating and sensitive account of the many upheavals accompanying this new form of knowledge and its attendant personal and ethical dilemmas. Like her sister, Alice Wexler has first-hand experience of the emotional ordeal (*épreuve*) and the anguish that comes with the status of being a person at risk of developing Huntington's disease. Alice and Nancy's mother began presenting symptoms in the 1950s and died from the disease in 1978. Hence, like her sister, Alice is not writing from a position of neutrality or indifference. Instead, she deploys her involvement with her subject matter as a convincing method for conducting historiographical and genealogical research.

Particular passages taken from her journals of the time, like those chronicling the period in 1983 when the indirect test was being developed, as well as the ensuing confusion, are particularly relevant to our current concerns. These passages reveal the extent to which both sisters had awaited this moment with impatience and even hope, one at the vanguard of medical research and the other from the vantage of historical inquiry. Yet in no less striking fashion, they also convey the veritable panic that takes hold as soon as such knowledge is at hand: "The immensity of it scares me shitless. The idea of really knowing – and what if it is 'positive'? Or if Nancy is? Once we know, there is no going back."[18]

So long as the existence of testing remained hypothetical, both sisters were convinced they would want to undergo it forthwith. Put directly, they were convinced

18 Wexler, *Mapping Fate*, 224.

they wanted to know. However, the situation was entirely different from the moment abstract hope became real option. Especially as it was now obvious that far, from addressing the test subject as an isolated individual, such a form of knowledge would strike their entire community, an inherently violent proposition:

> Dad says he's quite happy with things as they are, he could live the rest of his life very content, feeling confident we don't have the illness. He told Diane (a 60 Minutes journalist) "What I have now is joyousness. If I knew they were free of the disease, I'd feel ecstasy. It's not that great a gain. But there's an immense difference between joy and discovering one of them carried the gene. It's not worth the gamble." Diane kept asking about the value of certainty, the importance of knowledge for its own sake. Nancy says, "Yes, I've always believed in knowledge for its own sake. And it is ironic that after working for precisely that, I'm now finding it much more complex than I ever thought it would be." Diane: "Did you think you'd take the test when the linkage was discovered?" Nancy: "Absolutely. Yes. I never doubted it. And now I'm not sure."[19]

For the Wexlers and other members of the Huntington's community, it turned out that a gulf stretched between the abstract idea of a person having the power to know some aspect of their future and the concrete possibility of accessing this knowledge. In fact, when the test did become available to the public, following organizing efforts by Huntington's associations themselves, only a small number of at-risk persons chose to take the opportunity

19 Ibid., 233. Only very recently, in March 2020, Nancy Wexler has revealed that she has indeed inherited the mutation in an interview published by the *New York Times*. See Denise Grady, "Haunted by a Gene," *New York Times*, March 10, 2020, https://www.nytimes.com/2020/03/10/health/huntingtons-disease-wexler.html.

and get tested.[20] This large-scale shift away from enthu-
siastic advocacy to limited use demonstrates unambiguously that the existence of the predictive test fundamentally transformed Huntington's disease.

Testing consisted of a new kind of foreknowledge that
simultaneously upset existing practices towards HD –
whether familiar, medical, or ethical – along with the
social relations held by those involved. Put differently,
it displaced them. In terms of users' family relations:
more or less explicit ways of bringing up the disease
had evolved over generations; with the advent of this
new machine for producing foreknowledge, these were
turned on their head. From a clinical perspective: the
three-act play of "diagnosis, treatment, and prognosis"
that normally frames the relationship between patient
and doctor cannot hold in this new context. The structure of this play rests upon the assumption that an open-
ended narrative exists, tends towards a positive outcome
and requires practiced elaboration. There's the rub. In the
script provided by predictive testing, when the result is
unfavorable the future comes to stand in for a narrative
with no exit. Its outcome is always necessarily negative.
Furthermore, by thus compromising the foundations of
the doctor/patient relationship, the existence of the indirect and then direct test displaces medical epistemology
itself. Finally, in ethical terms, this new kind of medical
foreknowledge calls for a radical rethinking. As discussed
later in the book, it demands that at least two of bioethics' core premises be examined anew: *autonomy* and *informed consent*.

20 While precise statistics remain sorely lacking, it can be said that in
the course of their lives at most 20 per cent of at-risk persons decide
to undergo the procedures required for conducting the test, and that
only a fraction of this group then follows through to complete the
test. See Novas, *Governing "Risky" Genes*, and Nikolas Rose and Carlos Novas, "Genetic Risk and the Birth of the Somatic Individual,"
Economy and Society 29, no. 4 (2000): 485–513.

Testing before Testing

Two fields emerged in the 1950s and '60s that would un-
lock a better understanding of Huntington's disease: neuroscience and molecular biology, following Watson and
Crick's elaboration of the double helix structure of DNA
in 1953. Both soon underwent spectacular development.
The first center for neurobiology was established at Harvard in 1966, followed by the Society for Neuroscience in
1968. These burgeoning institutions and networks fos-
tered a promising new angle of research into neurotransmitters. Neurotransmitters are chemical substances such
as dopamine, serotonin, and endorphins sent from one
nerve cell to another. Evidence began to show that, depending on their quantity and quality, they could accel-
erate or block intercellular electrical messaging.

During this period, research into the neurotransmitters involved in Parkinson's disease demonstrated that
when the condition developed in patients their brains
concurrently displayed a fall in dopamine release. Because dopamine is an excitatory neurotransmitter its
absence would account for a range of Parkinson's symptoms including shaking, rigidity, and difficulty initiating
movement. Simply replacing patients' lack of dopamine
by way of synthetic dopamine injections proved inef-
fective. Evidently, the chemical substance was unable to
cross the blood-brain barrier. However, an intermediary
dopamine substance that would come to be known as
L-Dopa proved to be an effective substitute as the body
would convert it into dopamine that the brain could then
metabolize:

> If the L-dopa is administered in high enough doses,
> it can lead to a dramatic reduction of the symptoms.
> From a catastrophic illness that is seriously debilitat-

ing and often fatal, Parkinson's became an illness that can be partially controlled, even if it cannot be cured.[21]

Neurologists then discovered that when they treated Parkinson's patients with too high a dose of L-Dopa they tended to present symptoms akin to those experienced by Huntington's patients.[22] Consequently, dopamine inhibitors gave some measure of control over HD's motor symptoms. As for whether Huntington's patients produced too much dopamine or were hypersensitive to it, the jury was out. Brain autopsies of deceased patients gave no indication that dopamine levels were higher than those of neurologically healthy individuals. Regardless, the clinical configuration mediating neurologists' simultaneous encounter with Parkinson's and Huntington's diseases gave rise to the idea that the two conditions shared a symmetrical relationship.

This inverse symmetry then prompted the hypothesis that would lead to HD's very first experimental predictive test (not to be mistaken for the aforementioned and largely forgotten indirect genetic linkage test). Put simply: "administering L-dopa to people at risk for Huntington's might produce chorea-like symptoms in those who actually carried the gene."[23] At the start of the 1970s, neurologists André Barbeau and Harold L. Klawans investigated this hypothesis in an experiment involving thirty persons at risk of but not yet manifesting HD symptoms and a control group of twenty-four persons who were not at risk. During the experiment, all subjects received high doses of L-Dopa. The result was that a third of at-risk subjects developed transitory symptoms of chorea,

21 Wexler, *Mapping Fate*, 28.
22 L-Dopa is the same substance that produced effects on patients suffering from "sleeping sickness" in the late 1960s, as Oliver Sacks recounts in the fascinating book *Awakenings* (New York: Harper Perennial, 1990).
23 Wexler, *Mapping Fate*, 99

while none of the control group did. Later in the decade, more limited experiments on the effects of L-Dopa were conducted on homozygotes (children with both parents from Huntington's families).

Barbeau and Klawans's experiment merits discussion in light of the debate surrounding its results published in the *British Journal of Medicine* in 1972. This debate was not just integral to the historical milieu in which the indirect genetic test emerged in 1983. In addition, the arguments dominating these discussions, along with the assumptions and value judgments they carry, were able to cast fresh light on the *Guidelines for the Molecular Genetics Predictive Test in Huntington's Disease,* whose first version was published in 1990.

By June of 1973, the *Hastings Center Report* published Michael Hemphill's response to the published results of Barbeau and Klawans's experiment in an article titled "Pretesting for Huntington's Disease: An Overview."[24] Hemphill began with criticism of perceived inaccuracies in the protocols used to convey experimental results to at-risk persons involved. When the L-Dopa triggered choreic movements "were [patients] told the disease was now inevitable?" And conversely, that they were "off the hook" when it didn't?[25] The centerpiece of the article is a list of arguments for and against the general availability of an invasive, predictive test derived from L-Dopa. In brief, the three arguments for the test – which he assumes his peers share – are as follows: first, if everyone who tested "positive" did not reproduce or were ["constrained from doing so"], the disease would only occur as the result of a novel and exceedingly rare mutation. Second, at-risk persons should not have to live with either false hope or uncertainty any longer than necessary.

---

24 Michael Hemphill, "Pretesting for Huntington's Disease: An Overview," *Hastings Center Report* 3, no. 3 (June 1973): 12–13.
25 Ibid., 13.

And third, "for ethicists" he remarks, placing himself at a remove from what is to come, "such knowledge would be regarded as good *per se* because it increases the carrier's humanity. An analogy to the state of lost innocence could be made – where one could previously act without full knowledge of the consequences and thus avoid responsibility, one is now given the necessary knowledge to act responsibly. Thus to some to be fully human is to be responsible in this sense."[26]

Hemphill then lists counterarguments. First, diagnosis can be justified in cases where effective therapy or prophylaxis is available – which is not the case for Huntington's disease. In such a view, knowing or not knowing makes no difference to reality. Second, the test is questionable in that it provides patients with premature knowledge of their symptoms at the level of *inner* experience. Third, confusion surrounds the psychological motivations of those opting for the test. Finally, test results may prompt obstacles for obtaining medical insurance as well as access to education and employment. Hemphill ends by calling for careful scrutiny of the implications of predictive testing for Huntington's prior to making it generally available. In his view, it is reasonable to worry that people will ask for the test in order to learn they have been spared and will be unable to cope with the opposite outcome: "ultimately, the question is one of minimizing suffering in a situation with very few alternatives to suffering. Our responsibility for the ethical issues at hand is to ensure that all the parameters for decision-making are explored and that human sensitivity is not blunted by our concern to assimilate data or diagnose disease."[27]

A few months later, in the September issue of the *Hastings Center Report,* Frank R. Freemon published a reply to Hemphill. Evidently appalled, he says: "It seems to me

26 Ibid.
27 Ibid.

[Hemphill's] rejection of early diagnosis and prognosis damns much of modern medicine."[28] Freemon contends that rejecting Barbeau & Klawans's experiment because of the ethical and psychological issues it brings to light is a case of throwing the baby out with the bathwater. By extension, entire areas of modern medical practice would be null and void for walking the very same ethical tightrope. This he simply cannot abide. Furthermore, he argues, Hemphill takes a widely held but mistaken view of medicine that overemphasizes its therapeutic role. He counters with the following: "[A]ctually the doctor's role as a counselor is just as important as his role as pharmacologist or surgeon. Accurate and early diagnosis is important because then we can give accurate prognosis."[29] The reader quickly learns, however, that in Freemon's view such a "counseling" capacity does not refer to a mutually beneficial exchange of insights among doctor and patient, but rather to a one-way street in which the doctor lectures the patient on what's what. According to him, unwitting patients and their loved ones, ill-informed by rumor and word of mouth, are "sometimes so terrified of the unknowns of the illness as to be virtually paralyzed with hysteria" and so need to be reassured if not hushed by doctors bearing prognoses that neither minimize nor dramatize the situation but offer up its objective assessment. According to Freemon, the doctor achieves this by, among other things, "always holding out a ray of hope, usually based on future research."[30] Staking your hopes on an uncertain future sits in stark contrast to ideas about self-determination or today's notions of "empowerment," wherein patients are capable of activity and activation through forms of collective commitment

---

28 Frank R. Freemon, "Pretesting for Huntington's Disease: Another View," *Hastings Center Report* 3, no. 4 (September 1973): 13.

29 Ibid.

30 Ibid.

to building strategies and tactics for living as well as possible with a diagnosed disease.

In effect, hope such as this sets up a strict separation between ignorant patients and knowledgeable doctors who can heal them, at least in theory. In so doing, the author perpetuates understandings of medicine and research as the only way of knowing disease. He never considers the possibility that sickness could be the result of a co-constructed and experimental exploration, forged from tips and techniques shared by doctors and patients alike, an exploration that can itself bring relief to the sick person. Far from it, the doctor's first responsibility according to Freemon is protecting their patients from the dangers of a "naïve" attitude: "an understanding and frank discussion allows the patient and his family to prepare for the future, to stop the endless rounds of specialist after specialist, and to minimize the patient's natural tendency to squander his resources on faith healers and charlatans."[31] Real hope should be placed in true science, even if its results don't quite yet exist. Only true science is authorized to heal for the "right reasons." The second part of this book will turn to the substantive genealogy of this proposition.

Well before 1983, debate over the possibility of a predictive test for Huntington's was underway. It presents two other striking features: enduring and ongoing depictions of the disease as a horror story, and frequently explicit recourse to eugenic arguments. Hemphill, for instance, writes that "in the late stages of dementia the patient presents the pitiful picture of the complete ruin of a human being."[32] While painting the horror in subtler hues, S. Thomas channels eugenicist ideology to even more devastating results in a 1982 article published in the *British Medical Journal*. He writes:

31 Ibid.
32 Hemphill, "Pretesting for Huntington's Disease," 12.

The distress and inefficiency of those counseled in the first stages of their illness make some of them incapable of using effective measures of birth control. On this view, as on the view that the urge and determination to procreate in the face of the possibility of the disease is almost a prodromal symptom of the disease itself, any reduction in family size as a result of counseling is likely to come preferentially from those who do not have the mutant gene.[33]

Not content to depict persons with HD as deeply irrational and lacking judgment, he charges them with a pathological urge to reproduce. He pinpoints this urge within a liminal phase of the condition lying between presymptomatic status and symptomatic onset. During this "prodromal" phase, patients are typically considered quite capable of good judgment. And of course, this argument only holds to the extent that "reduction in family size" – a sophisticated turn of phrase that obfuscates a fundamentally eugenic position – has been agreed upon as a moral norm. To be sure, the need for such a reduction comes across as especially convincing when Huntington's disease is simply, simultaneously, and unequivocally demonized. At the time such views, albeit implicitly eugenic for all intents and purposes, were evidently acceptable, at least when it came to HD, as reflected in these recommendations from Husquinet, Franck, and Vranckx concerning L-Dopa experiments on monozygotic twins published in 1973:

We would add that a prediction test is useful only for those who have to choose between marriage and celibacy, procreation or interruption of the line of descendants, since no preventive medical treatment can

33 S. Thomas, "Ethics of a Predictive Test for Huntington's Chorea," *British Medical Journal* 284, no. 6326 (May 1982): 1383–85.

yet be recommended to potential choreic individuals. Bearing this in mind, application of the test to a 50 year old woman seems useless.[34]

Guidelines

But prophetic speech announces an impossible future, or makes the future it announces, because it announces it, something impossible, a future one would not know how to live and that must upset all the sure givens of existence. When speech becomes prophetic, it is not the future that is given, it is the present that is taken away, and with it any possibility of a firm, stable, lasting presence.
– Maurice Blanchot[35]

In 1983, before completion of the first phase of research into the genetic marker for Huntington's disease, debate surrounded the possible risks and consequences flowing from wider availability of a predictive test for the condition. The advent of indirect genetic testing as a real possibility launched a phase of more or less (un)controlled use in the shape of clinical studies aimed at assessing the test's reliability. The resulting situation soon led doctors and representatives of the Huntington's community to the conclusion that recommendations for the use of testing were needed. The initial version of these collectively designed recommendations appeared in 1990, published in quick succession in the *Journal of Medical Genetics* and *Neurology*.[36] They were re-edited with minor revisions in

---

34 H. Husquinet, G. Franck, and C. Vranckx, "Detection of Future Cases of Huntington's Chorea by the L-dopa Load Test: Experiment with Two Monozygotic Twins," *Advances in Neurology* 1 (1973): 301–10.

35 Maurice Blanchot, *The Book to Come*, trans. Charlotte Mandell (Stanford: Stanford University Press, 2003), 79.

36 "Ethical Issues Policy Statement on Huntington's Disease Molecular Genetics Predictive Test," *Journal of the Neurological Sciences* 94, nos. 1–3 (1989): 327–32, and *Journal of Medical Genetics* 27, no. 7 (1990): 34–38.

1994, in response to the arrival of the direct test.[37] The decision to formalize such recommendations was made during conferences of the International Huntington Association and the World Federation of Neurology in the French city of Lille in 1985; the first version was tabled four years later in Vancouver in July 1989. The "Guidelines for the Molecular Genetics Predictive Test in Huntington's Disease" were intended to provide "recommendations concerning the use of a predictive test for the early detection of Huntington's disease"[38] As signaled in the introduction in 1990, they aimed at establishing "realistic, ethical principles based on current knowledge and techniques in molecular genetics" in order to "govern the application of the predictive test" and "protect at risk subjects."[39] The first revision in 1994 added a new item: "the guidelines are also intended to assist clinicians, geneticists, and ethics committees as well as lay organizations [i.e., user groups] to resolve difficulties arising from the application of the test."[40] Considering that the L-Dopa testing debate had set the stage, it follows that, above all, the guidelines also endeavored to limit the damage caused by a discursive milieu dominated by eugenic ideology.

The "Guidelines" are divided into nine sections each containing their own sub-sections, with the document split into two columns, recommendations on the left and related comments on the right. Aside from adjustments

---

37 "Guidelines for the Molecular Genetics Predictive Test in Huntington's Disease," *Neurology* 44, no. 8 (1994): 1533–36, and *Journal of Medical Genetics* 31, no. 7 (1994): 555–59. An updated version published in 2013 did not introduce any major changes. See "Recommendations for the Predictive Genetic Test in Huntington's Disease," *Clinical Genetics* 83, no. 3 (2013): 221–31.

38 "Ethical Issues Policy Statement on Huntington's Disease Molecular Genetics Predictive Test," *Journal of Medical Genetics*, 34.

39 Ibid.

40 "Guidelines for the Molecular Genetics Predictive Test in Huntington's Disease," *Journal of Medical Genetics*, 555.

to the order of the text and new data regarding the discovery of the exact location of the Huntington's gene, the language remains more or less consistent in all versions.[41] In particular, the guidelines give a precise definition of who testing is available for, and when and under what conditions. They also suggest a set of roles and functions that should arise in the overall course of testing, in other words, before, during, and after the genetic test itself. The first recommendation is short: "All persons who may wish to take the test should be given up to date, relevant information so that they can make an informed, voluntary decision" (555). The second one stipulates that "[t]he decision to take the test is the sole choice of the person concerned" (ibid.) and that only those having reached the age of majority have the right to take the test – with the exception of prenatal testing. Hence, from the outset the authors draw upon the principles of patient autonomy, the right to know (or not to know), and informed consent, all fundamental to the ethics of medicine as it emerged in the United States during the 1960s and 1970s. They also elevate another principle: "Persons should not be discriminated against in any way as a result of genetic testing for Huntington's disease" (556). A further recommendation calls for specially trained "counselors" to accompany persons throughout the testing process. They are to be fully-fledged members of multidisciplinary teams that include geneticists, neurologists, social workers, psychiatrists, and specialists in medical ethics. In addition to these roles, at-risk persons have the option of nominating a "companion" to accompany them throughout all stages of the process. Sections three and four describe the counselor's role within this constellation of actors. "The counselling unit should plan with

---

41 Hereafter, I will refer to the 1994 version, which is used to this day, as printed in the *Journal of Medical Genetics*. Page references are given between parentheses in the main text.

the participant a follow up protocol which provides for support during the pre- and post-test stages, whether or not a person chooses a companion" (ibid.). Moreover, the counselor is responsible for recommending the participant touch base with a local Huntington's association and for explaining, in concert with the medical team, the technical aspects of the test as well as the ongoing lack of either prevention or cure for the disease. There is explicit language indicating that this discussion must include "information on alternatives the applicant can adopt," such as the possibility "[n]ot to take the test for the time being" (558). Sections six and seven are less relevant to the present analysis; they cover the possible need for preliminary neurological testing along with pre-natal diagnosis. Section eight, however, is significant. Under the heading "The Test and Delivery of Results" (559) it stipulates that prospective test participants must heed a minimum waiting period of one month between initial consultation and the decision to take the test. It also insists that once participants undertake the test, they must receive the results as soon as possible at a time set up in advance: "The manner in which the results will be delivered should be discussed between the counselling team and the person" (559). Finally, the ninth section states that in the post-testing period, the counselor should keep in regular contact with the test participant for a minimum of one month. During this time, lay organizations should also expect to play an important role.

Hence, the "Guidelines" are a response to the many psychological, generational, ethical, economic, and public health questions brought about by the existence of predictive testing for HD. To this day, at least in the United States and in Europe, they continue to provide a common orientation for the clinical organization of testing procedures. Nonetheless, exactly how they are applied in concrete terms, within a variety of institutions and across different health systems, depends on a whole set of parameters. The most decisive of these is the question of who takes on which of the roles designated in the guidelines – particularly that of the counselor – not simply at the level of the individual but also at the level of their disciplinary affiliation. Much like the staging of a play, interpretation therefore varies from country to country and institution to institution.

In a French clinic in the mid-2000s, Alice Rivières found herself exposed to a performance of the guidelines that was truly devastating, as clearly rendered in her *Manifesto*. It was as if the whole process was stuck in a routine. Among the multidisciplinary team, the psychologist appointed to the role of the counselor appeared to be there not to offer support but provide an assessment based on strict criteria of whether Alice would be able to receive a potentially adverse test result:[42] "[the psychologist responds] that I appear quite unemotional, that I should let my feelings out."[43] Along with the rest of the multidisciplinary team, Alice ends up dealing with throughout the process, the psychologist conveys the following sense to her:

> It feels like a driving test: I have to prove who I am, they have to think I'm strong enough to quell their fears that I'll kill myself because of them, yet I also have to appear upset enough not to come across as emotionally shut down. It's a tricky line to walk, but I end up pulling it off and they allow me to get my results two months after the start of the testing process, the hallmark of a successful applicant. They draw two

42 This kind of assessment largely serves to allow medicine to insure itself against its own transformative power. In such circumstances, the object of assessment is above all the likelihood that the person seeking to know their genetic status could commit suicide.

43 Rivières, "The Dingdingdong Manifesto," 25.

vials of blood, because the results have to be double-checked by two different labs.[44]

On the day she learns of the result, she does not go alone but rather, as advised, accompanied by her two closest friends. Her account of this day speaks volumes: the neurologist

delivers the sentence as my CAG number (CAG stands for Cytosine-Adenine-Guanine. More than 36 repeats of this glutamine on the 4th chromosome indicate the presence of the gene responsible for Huntington's disease): 44. No need for a second opinion. [...] She then turns to [Alice's friend] Emmanuelle and tells her how dreadful it will be for family and friends, and that she needs to quickly start getting help herself. Not content with cursing me, she dunks my friends in her pox as well.[45]

What emerges from Alice's retelling is that the real injury does not stem from the sole reference to a CAG count of 44, and thus the unequivocal fact that she bears the mutation, inherited from her mother, herself at an advanced stage of the disease, which she inherited from her father, who inherited it from his mother, and so on. Rather, the violence prominently resides in the gestures and sentences surrounding this information. The doctor turns away from her to turn toward the friend accompanying her, in order to inform her of the unbearable nature of the coming situation, for Alice along with all of her loved ones. The veritable curse is not – or at least not exclusively – to be found in the fact that Alice inherited the "bad" gene, but rather in the fact that next to this definitive prognosis lies another one entirely, one that would

44 Ibid.
45 Ibid., 27–28.

define or prescribe in equally absolute terms exactly how this legacy will come to pass. The future has already happened. The gene's effects will simply be destructive and catastrophic. They will diminish her little by little. There is nothing that can be done about this because at the end of the day, at least for now, there is no treatment available for Huntington's patients. The radical and ravaging violence of this situation of diagnostic and predictive prophesying is contained in the utterance of a total inability to act: "The test is a destiny-making machine. Going through with it means witnessing the radical and immediate transformation of your inner truth, that constantly quivering kaleidoscope, into the simple truth of a medical definition."[46] Diagnostic situations like this one, at least when they are conducted in this way, effectively give those involved the idea that when the result is "positive," there's only one thing left to do: wait for the beginning of the end. Instead of uncertainty or a puzzle needing to be worked through together, the only thing on the table is acceptance in the face of certain disaster. Well before the first signs of any symptoms emerge, the person now tested becomes a *patient* in a literal sense, a suffering person who can only wait in patience.

To be sure, this particular story of diagnosis and its fateful character cannot be generalized. It does, however, highlight the danger of transforming international recommendations into institutionally reified routines, which is to say, into processes that are neither up for discussion nor negotiation by their very participants. What is in danger, properly speaking, is the truth of a disease and its diagnosis alongside the ability of people to function psychosocially, the very same people said to enjoy autonomy, informed consent and the right to know. The tragedy of the process, as Alice Rivières recounts it and which culminates in the disclosure of the result, lies in

46 Ibid., 28.

how, once endless, the many forms a life can get win-nowed down to a single one. Moreover, the form that life then takes is a cruel and hopeless one; it becomes binding and nobody can influence it in any way – not the doc-tor, not the tested person and not their loved ones. This kind of medical truth, bearing no therapeutic knowledge and yet presenting itself as the sole legitimate author-ity over disease, is freighted with a particular kind of vio-lence. This violence, says Alice, stems from the fact that, in spite of its own inability to act, medicine claims the authority to crush any and all other possible truths.

Alice's story places us before a distinctly *problematic* situation. While inviting rigorous and in-depth analysis, this situation throws up an initial temptation to rush to judgment and unreservedly denounce the medical estab-lishment, its associated disciplines, and their practition-ers. The real challenge this situation and others like it raise is, I submit, to go one step further and interrogate the propositional potential of conceptual, historical, and empirical research itself. To put things somewhat more modestly: can we interrogate the resources such research provides for moving past a standstill, for learning not to complain about difficult and unbearable situations but to take them as a starting point for constructing well-articulated problems? If so, what does a "well-articulated problem" look like, and what kind of problematization might be tailored to welcoming this new kind of fore-knowledge?

2

Exploratory Sites

A New Species Called the Test;
Or, How to Construct a Problem

> *Oh, Frankenstein, be not equitable to every other, and trample*
> *upon me alone, to whom thy justice, and even thy clemency and*
> *affection, is most due. Remember that I am thy creature; I ought to*
> *be thy Adam; but I am rather the fallen angel, whom thou drivest*
> *from joy for no misdeed. [...] You, my creator, abhor me; what hope*
> *can I gather from your fellow-creatures, who owe me nothing?*
> —Mary Shelley[1]

"A problem does not exist, apart from its solutions. Far from disappearing in this overlay, however, it insists and persists in these solutions. A problem is determined at the same time as it is solved," writes Deleuze drawing on the philosophy of Henri Bergson.[2] Problem and solution coexist according to this logic, even though the one does not envelop the other and cannot be reduced to it either. "[The problem's] determination is not the same as its solution: the two elements differ in kind, the deter-

---

1   Mary Shelley, *Frankenstein; or, The Modern Prometheus* (Boston: Sever, Francis, & Co., 1869), 78–79.

2   Gilles Deleuze, *Difference and Repetition*, trans. Paul Patton (London and New York: Continuum, 1994), 163.

mination amounting to the genesis of the concomitant solution."[3] Taking Deleuze's proposition seriously, it follows that there is no such thing as a problem without a solution. In other words, a problem only warrants the name "problem" when it is well constructed, which is to say, constructed with a view to a solution. When a problem can exist beyond solution, he refers to it, following Bergson, as a "false problem." Bergson and Deleuze both insist that the role of philosophy is not to suffer (*subir*) a problem "as it is posited by language."[4] For, as Bergson puts it, if philosophy was, in truth, nothing other than the repetition of predetermined problems then it would be

> condemned in advance to receive a ready-made solution or, at best, simply to choose between the two or three only possible solutions, which are co-eternal to this positing of the problem. One might just as well say that all truth is already virtually known [...] and that philosophy is a jigsaw puzzle where the task is to construct with the pieces society gives us the design it is unwilling to show us. One might just as well assign to the philosopher the role and the attitude of the schoolboy, who seeks the solution persuaded that if he had the boldness to risk a glance at the master's book, he would find it there, set down opposite the question. But the truth is that in philosophy and even elsewhere it is a question of finding the problem and consequently of positing it, even more than of solving it.[5]

Bergson and Deleuze therefore enjoin us to trust in the capacity of thought – not so much to respond to prob-

---

3 Ibid.
4 Henri Bergson, *The Creative Mind: An Introduction to Metaphysics*, trans. Mabelle Andison (Mineola: Dover Publications, 2007), 51.
5 Ibid.

lems existing prior to it, but to participate in producing new possibles, insofar as constructing good problems shifts and revitalizes reality. Consequently, no matter how difficult and unbearable it may be, a situation is no more a problem than a question is. Indeed, when positing a question or confronting a situation, we depend entirely upon reality as it presents itself to us. To move beyond the question/situation as given, and beyond its mere critique as well, and to shift into an active force with which we might intervene into reality, it will not do to simply glance at the master's book – for there is no answer sheet drawn up ahead of time. The work of problem construction can instead be compared with landscape painting, the staging of a play, or storytelling; these practices, in positioning (*posant*) various elements, write them into relations of inclusion and exclusion or influence and causality, and thereby compose (*composent*) newly arranged (*disposés*) spaces in which to act.[6]

When it comes to Huntington's disease, it may be that medicine focuses on a false problem, a "distressing and insoluble"[7] problem: incurability. Its primary concern is therefore its own inability to act as a curative art towards the disease, which is to say, a situation that, for the time being at any rate, admits no solution. The falsity of the problem results from placing the "curable" in contradistinction to the "incurable." Medical solutions, according to common understanding, must be therapeutic in kind or, for chronic diseases, at the very least resemble treatment. When this is lacking, "we work our way backwards from one cause to another; if we stop somewhere along the way, it is not because our intelligence seeks nothing further beyond, it is because our imagination ends

---

6   See Claude de Jonckheere, *83 mots pour penser l'intervention en travail social* (Geneva: Éditions IES, 2010), 321–24.

7   Bergson, *The Creative Mind,* 64.

up averting its gaze, as though from an abyss, to avoid dizziness."[8]

To help clarify why we must open the imagination and our other senses in order to construct an otherwise insoluble and dizzying problem/solution well, consider the so-called "camel problem." This story has intrigued many thinkers,[9] including two of Dingdingdong's founding members, Vinciane Despret and Isabelle Stengers. It is of particular pertinence to a disease that centers questions of heredity.

Before his death, the desert prince Ali decides to bequeath his pack of seventeen camels to his three sons. But to this inheritance he hitches a riddle: half the bequest will go to the eldest, a third to the middle son, and a ninth to the youngest. Before saying his final goodbyes, Ali makes his sons promise not to kill any of the animals and to share them out through strictly peaceful means. Ali dies and his sons find themselves faced with an impossible division; a struggle over succession seems inevitable. The three sons therefore seek out a wise man from the neighboring village and ask him for advice. He says to them: "I cannot solve the problem. All I can do is give you my camel. He is old, skinny, and not very brave, but he will help you share out your inheritance." And so the three brothers find themselves with eighteen camels: the oldest takes half, or nine of them, the middle son a third, or six, and the youngest a ninth, or two – and they return the remaining camel to the wise man.

The father left his sons with neither a vast fortune nor a simple and humble inheritance; he left them with a riddle (*énigme*). The riddle is not of a strictly mathemati-

8 Ibid. Translation modified.
9 See Pierre Ageron, "Le partage des dix-sept chameaux et autres arithmétiques attributes à l'immam 'Alî: Mouvance et circulation de récits de la tradition musulmane chiite," *Revue d'histoire des mathématiques* 19 (2013): 1–41, https://ageron.users.lmno.cnrs.fr/17chameaux.pdf.

cal nature. It also summons them to think through what they can do with what they have been given. They must prove themselves worthy of the confidence their father placed in them by leaving them with something they would have to construct. Only upon doing so will they be able to claim their inheritance. Thus, what is at stake here is to construct a fertile milieu for the bequest and to do so without cheating. The sons do not simply inherit seventeen camels, as these are rather the vehicle and the outcome of an inheritance that simultaneously – thanks to the eighteenth camel – transforms itself into a problem.[10] Hence, they do not pull off this transformation all by themselves. When they open up to the wise man, when they socialize their complicated situation by confiding in an outside party who can add something to the family arrangement, only then are they able to become their father's heirs.

Problems aren't just out there; they don't come ready-made. To the contrary, constructing a problem takes careful and creative work whose outcome – the problem itself – bestows all actors implicated or involved with the ability to act on it. This is the sense in which a problem's construction and solution always go together. Although lacking concrete or defined contours, it is a solution, as it were, that orients all work on a problem and secures commitment from those it gathers together.

If effective therapeutic or prophylactic treatments for HD had become available at the same time as the genetic knowledge behind predictive testing, then some kind of balance between medical theory and practice would no doubt have been found, as has been the case with multiple sclerosis in recent decades. Yet because of therapeutic non-knowledge in the case of Huntington's disease,

10 I am largely indebted to Vinciane Despret for this rereading of the riddle. Cf. *Our Emotional Makeup: Ethnopsychology and Selfhood,* trans. Marjolijn de Jager (New York: Other Press, 2004).

things turned out differently. Rather than just a passing phase or a side effect, predictive testing has come to dominate the frame since the 1980s, to the point of becoming a force of its own. By 2000, Nancy Wexler came to speak of the test with lingering apprehension: "sometimes I ask myself what sort of creature we've put into the world."[11]

Taking heed of Wexler's choice of words means reckoning with predictive testing as a new creature, a being to be added to conventional forms of epistemological and ethical know-how, one whose presence dares these forms of knowledge and practice to transform themselves. As when a new, hitherto unknown species appears within a biological milieu, involving this creature in the construction of well-posited problems means adopting an ecological perspective. As with ecosystem ecology, an ecology of diagnosis is tasked with "questions of process, namely, those likely to include disparate terms. Ecology can and should, for example, take into account the consequences, for a given milieu, of the appearance of a new technical practice just as it does for the consequences of climate change or the appearance of a new species."[12]

In order to approach predictive testing for HD as the ecologist would a new species emerging within different ecosystems or milieus (the family, clinical practice, ethics), which is to say by taking the measure of the ensuing consequences, the formation of these same milieus must first be reconstructed. Such a historical perspective helps draw into view the kinds (*espèces*) of practices and concepts that this test-creature displays and displaces.

11 In interview with Swiss science journalist Reto U. Schneider, first published in *NZZ-Folio* and available here: Reto Schneider, "Wissen ist Ohnmacht," *Die Zeit*, October 12, 2000, https://www.zeit.de/2000/42/Wissen_ist_Ohnmacht. Translation and emphasis mine.

12 Isabelle Stengers, *Cosmopolitics I*, trans. Robert Bononno (Minneapolis: University of Minnesota Press, 2010), 33. The following reflections on an ecology of practices are crucially inspired by Stengers's work.

It aims at acquiring an understanding of the values and modes of evaluation and meaning making of these practices and concepts, by accounting for the ways in which they matter to someone speaking and acting in their name. In this sense, thinking through practices ecologically presents neither the prospect of judgment (grounded in general hypotheses, at a remove from the world of facts and values proper to the practice at hand) nor of tolerance (wherein "anything goes"). Rather, the ecologist's task when considering a given practice is to take its requirements and obligations seriously, to recognize its value and perhaps even to evaluate it accordingly – not on the basis of general ideals of rationality, thereby dismissing what counts for the practice itself.

The picture of diagnosis given by Alice Rivières is indisputably ruinous; it is tempting to hold medicine alone responsible, or more specifically those medical practitioners directly involved. The ecological point of view presents the distinct advantage of forcing a moment's pause, producing an interruption, and calling for a closer look in lieu of hastily offered judgment (or blame). It dares the critic to approach the creature, treading ever so carefully, and to take up the many perspectives of all actors present (and of their practices) – namely those for whom, in one way or another, the creature matters.

Thus, the creature's particular, unruly features become open to questioning. What is there to it that so disturbs otherwise well-honed forms of knowledge and practice? What would it take to fabricate a milieu worthy of a diagnosis such as this, namely one with the necessary primers with which those involved (doctors, caregivers, patients, and loved ones) might shift from a position of powerlessness to one of active problem construction? How to cultivate an ecology of diagnosis that could place all actors involved in situations where they become capable of acting to the fullest extent possible?

Reprise

So begins the search for camels, camels that will contribute something to the milieu of the creature known as the predictive test for HD, something with which to welcome it, to learn to love and foster it and, at the same time, to tame it. Such camels will have a constructive purpose, one that does not amount to damage control, to curbing the test's destructive power once the deed is done and the results are in. Instead, it involves reorganizing this entity's milieu with a view to the future.

Where might such creatures be found? They tend to be hard to retrieve, dwelling in remote places. In order to investigate this unfamiliar field with its many nooks and crannies, it will be helpful to anchor the thread of my investigation on a strategic pivot, unfurling it behind me as I go so as to always remain in a position to return to my initial point of departure. I will take the moment Alice Rivières learned of her test results as this anchor point, taking it to be an exemplary scene whose milieu is made from the stuff of modern medicine:

> She delivers the sentence as my CAG number: 44. No need for a second opinion. The number is well above the threshold that separates those carrying the disease from those who do not. She then turns to Emmanuelle and tells her how dreadful it will be for family and friends, and that she needs to quickly start getting help herself.[13]

The "pure" genetic information hidden beneath the number 44 indicates the following: forty-four repeats of the DNA sequence are to be found on the small arm of Alice's fourth chromosome and this, to be specific, at the location of the gene for Huntington's disease. Accord-

13   Alice Rivières, "The Dingdingdong Manifesto," this volume, 27.

ingly, this means she carries the disease. The three persons present all share this knowledge; it needs no further explanation. What happens next, with a simple gesture and without shift in register, when the neurologist turns away from Alice, towards Emmanuelle, announces that things will become unbearable for everyone involved, and counsels them to seek help immediately, actually *converts* genetic information about Alice's status as a carrier into an announcement regarding this same status's coming effects. This conflates "44" as genetic information and the lived experience of HD's symptoms, as if these belonged to the same order of factual, invariable knowledge whereas, in reality, both the onset and experience of HD's symptoms vary widely on a case-by-case basis. Hence the bequest being made is neither given nor received as a riddle, as something leaving open the manner and means with which those involved are to claim and cultivate it. Instead, the number 44 takes the form of a curse presaging cruel consequences.

The distinction between performative and constative utterances, owed to the British philosopher and founder of speech act theory John L. Austin, is particularly helpful for making sense of this situation. In Austin's view, what characterizes a constative utterance is that it names something essentially verifiable. Accordingly "when referring to the future, the statement becomes a prognosis. [...] By contrast, a performative utterance, although it also reports something, is neither verifiable nor temporally identifiable."[14] In *doing* something rather than just *saying* something, what defines a performative speech act is that "the issuing of the utterance is the performing of an action."[15] Performative utterances are neither true nor

14 Herbert Marks, "Der Geist Samuels. Die biblische Kritik an prognostischer Prophetie," in *Prophetie und Prognostik*, eds. Daniel Weidner and Stefan Willer (Berlin: Fink, 2013), 99–121. Translation mine.
15 John L. Austin, *How to Do Things with Words* (Oxford: Oxford University Press, 1962), 6.

false but rather successful and unsuccessful, or as Austin puts it "happy" and "unhappy."[16] Whereas a constative speech act accounts for a reality independent of itself, a performative speech act does not. No doubt the most well known performative is the sentence "I now pronounce you husband and wife," which, when announced by a priest or civil servant, is immediately and simultaneously accompanied by the transformation of its addressees into spouses. When it comes to the announcement addressed to Alice Rivières, a surreptitious confusion takes place between these two types of fundamentally distinct utterances. In light of this ambiguity, some measure of control should obtain over the performative power of diagnostic-constative speech that runs the risk, at least in the context in question, of becoming a self-fulfilling prophecy.

The danger of the power of prophetic speech is perhaps most plainly revealed in a passage in the Old Testament. The Book of Jeremiah focuses on the question of the difference between true and false prophecy. Jeremiah announces to Hananiah that he shall die: "Therefore thus says the Lord; Behold I will cast you off the face of the earth: this year you shall die."[17] Two months later, Hananiah dies. For this reason, writes the comparative literature scholar Herbert Marks, Jeremiah's prophecy at first appears to be a "prognostic prophecy."[18] Such a prophecy reports (*constate*) something ahead of time, that will happen no matter what and of which only God's emissary can have foreknowledge:

> Upon further consideration, however, it appears that what Jeremiah puts on display is less his informed knowledge of the future than his linguistic superi-

16 Ibid., 14.
17 *New King James Version*, Jer 28:16.
18 Marks, "Der Geist Samuels," 105. Translation mine.

ority. For it is unclear whether Hananiah would still have died had Jeremiah not announced his prophecy. [...] The prophecy is already fulfilled in and through words that relate to Hananiah personally, words that Jeremiah does not so much address to but rather aim at Hananiah. Uttering them means immediately enacting them.[19]

For *prophets* not only speak of the future, evoking that which comes *ahead* (*pro*), they also speak *for* (*pro*) or in the name of someone or something, whether a divine power or science itself, that authorizes and legitimates their speech.

It is possible to decry the manifestly hapless communication skills of the doctor facing Alice Rivières, to denounce and to criticize this medical practitioner, and thereby explain this diagnostic situation's failure as a matter of personal shortcomings. Instead, I would like to offer a symptomatic reading of the situation that attempts, carefully and precisely, to take into account the regimes of knowledge and information governing it. The gesture of turning away from Alice indicates a shift, or at least the potential for a shift, from constative speech ("44") to performative speech. Unlike Jeremiah (who knows that he speaks in God's name and can therefore trust in the performative power of his utterance), the practitioner is seized by a professional duty to provide "objective" information to their interlocutors and so slips surreptitiously into the performative register.

The vocational literature written by and for doctors, which I have mentioned earlier, confirms the habitual nature of such poor judgment when it comes to distinguishing between registers. From *Breaking Bad News* to *The Difficult Conversation*, these publications all present a blind spot that, I submit, stymies the ability of practitioners

19 Ibid., 107. Translation mine.

to reflect upon their own practice. Briefly put, it is the implicit assumption that the knowledge awaiting communication is made up of fundamentally neutral facts, even though these have undeniably value-laden effects. This assumption presupposes that diagnosis is appropriately expressed in constative speech acts. Currently contained in guidelines as well as legal and ethical obligations surrounding informed consent, the patient's right to know follows the same logic. It assumes that doctors are in possession of diagnostic knowledge, a quintessentially neutral thing and the objective product of science, something that their patients are to receive unaltered, accompanied if need be with information about different treatment options.[20] Of course this does not mean that the way in which these facts are communicated makes no difference. On the contrary, doctors are required to demonstrate empathy, sensitivity, and attentiveness to patients when delivering such information. But when it comes to dangers haunting this scene other than objective facts, responsibility falls upon a practitioner's psyche or, to be precise, their psychological aptitude. Medicine itself is relieved of these troublesome companions. In fact, when diagnoses are viewed as information, which is to say as neutral entities, and when they are treated as such in practice, then the only appreciable difference lies in the individual skill required to communicate them, which varies greatly from doctor to doctor. To be sure, there is wide recognition today of the need to learn (or relearn) a form of closeness with patients or to adopt an empathic attitude and approach. Indeed, efforts a re made to teach these qualities to medical students, e.g., through pedagogical role-playing games. Notwithstand-

---

20 Such thinking reflects the modern separation of sick person and disease that physician and philosopher Georges Canguilhem describes as the foundational gesture of medicine as a scientific discipline. Cf. *Writings on Medicine*, trans. Stefanos Geroulanos and Todd Meyers (New York: Fordham University Press, 2012).

ing these good intentions, to me this seems to be more a consolation than a veritable desire to *push thinking further*, as Alice might say, through situated encounters. This will no doubt remain so, so long as medicine holds firm to an understanding of knowledge borrowed from physics and chemistry and continues, moreover, to model itself upon them.

In view of this, it is no longer sufficient to attribute to psychological ineptitude the way in which Alice's doctor collapses, in one fell swoop, genetic information and its attendant terrifying storyline. In light of a range of features central to the history of modern medicine and to the history of diagnosis, this gesture proves to be riddled with a series of assumptions that have become implicit. By deciding to analyze and read this scene from an historical perspective, I am in no way seeking to justify or downplay the behavior of this particular doctor in this particular situation. Rather, I am committed to thinking about such behavior as the expression of particular operations foundational to the production of modern medical knowledge that, having come to pass as natural and self-evident, risk vanishing from view.

First Site: Separating the Sick Person from the Disease

"With an efficacy we cannot but appreciate," writes Georges Canguilhem, whose writings on the history of medicine orient the coming discussion, "contemporary medicine is founded on the progressive dissociation of disease and the sick person, seeking to characterize the sick person by the disease, rather than identify a disease on the basis of the bundle of symptoms spontaneously presented by the patient."[21] More specifically, what began as a heuristic dissociation of disease and the sick person in the name of diagnostic and therapeutic method cul-

21 Ibid., 35. Translation modified.

minated in an impersonal way of identifying patients. A telling expression of this is the manner in which doctors readily speak to one another about "the pneumonia case in room 12" or "the appendicitis op in the recovery theater." There is nothing self-evident about this dissociation, so how did it come to be? Premodern medicine and its attendant conceptualizations of disease addressed sick people in their singularity. The symptoms of the latter guided the methods of the former – whether diagnostic or therapeutic. In its endeavors to become a science, however, modern medicine gradually reorganized itself around the central aim of defining, naming, and categorizing diseases as stable entities that, by consequence, were relatively independent of the sick person.

When medicine strove to become a science like any other, diseases became entities endowed with a life of their own and with a relatively independent mode of existence when it came to the bodies let alone the persons they affected. Under these conditions, the universalizing claims of medical knowledge gained a foothold. Meanwhile, each patient became a case in the proper sense of the word, the grounds for deducing universal truths, specifically, the objective nature and clinical course of such and such a disease – its natural history. Once a disease was described as unambiguously and comprehensively as could be, its definition meant it could be recognized from its symptoms and its signs. Conversely, as new cases gave rise to new findings, these definitions could be further extended, refined, and sometimes refuted.

Over time and to this day, people within the medical field itself have repeatedly spoken out and questioned whether medicine is consistent with a model of knowledge production borrowed from physics and chemistry. Historian of science Charles Rosenberg explains that in 1827 the physician John Robertson remarks: "whether a nosological arrangement, the fruit of modern pathology, is a hopeless expectation, remains yet to be seen."[22] He goes on, "the degree to which diseases are modified by constitution, season, climate, and an infinite variety of accidental circumstances, renders it at least doubtful." Such a view, however, did gain traction. By according lesser significance to the influence of the environment, to a disease's many milieus, or to the singularities of its manifestation in a given organism, person, place, and so on, medicine staked its success on the pivotal role of accurate and independent etiology and nosology. As early as 1804, British doctor Thomas Trotter argued that "the name and definition of a disease are perhaps of more importance than is generally thought. They are like a central point to which converging rays tend: they direct future inquirers how to compare facts, and become, as it were, the base on which accumulating knowledge is to be heaped."[23]

However, composing and ascribing these names and definitions could only happen from a base of clear clinical signs, identified as causes, and with corresponding diagnostic methods. Directly cast in the image of physical and chemical experiments, they were meant to be of universal value, independent of space and time, of the experimental personnel involved, or of doctors and their patients. This implied the development of methods and technologies that could push doctors' subjective determinations into the background and limit patients' insights to mere suggestions, rather than allowing them a central role in knowledge-making. Patients were to be regarded as objects and doctors were to adopt a distanced attitude, like experimenters in a laboratory, earning them the credibility owed to the producer of neutral and autonomous facts.

22 Charles E. Rosenberg, *Our Present Complaint* (Baltimore: Johns Hopkins University Press: 2007), 17.
23 Cited in ibid.

Since Galileo's time, if not before, a distanced attitude is constitutive of the modern definition of the irrefutable scientific experiment. Indeed, the moment at which the experimenter withdraws from the experimental apparatus she has designed is a crucial one. This move authorizes the experiment to become a truthful event. Withdrawal also serves to demonstrate that the experiment's success in no way requires the experimenting person – nature must speak for herself.[24]

As soon as the diagnostic and therapeutic process submits to this scientific ideal of neutrality, the doctor takes up the role of the *experimenter* in the strict sense of the word. She must therefore make herself as transparent as possible in relation to the object being examined. Although she may be the one who sets up a particular knowledge apparatus (by prescribing a drug, for instance), she soon withdraws to wait and observe. With this same move, the patient is transformed into a piece of nature. It is her body that speaks for her, expressing the drug's effects in the form of visualizations generated continuously by various measuring devices – cardiograms, blood pressure readings, and respiratory frequencies.

Instead of the patients and their experiences of suffering, what lies at the center of such an approach are the entities that diseases have become, with their own functional mechanisms and ways of responding to therapeutic alternatives for overcoming them. As Canguilhem writes:

Disease refers to medicine rather than to evil. When a doctor speaks of Basedow's disease (that is, of goiter exophthalmia), he designates a state of endocrine dysfunction whose presentation of symptoms, etiological diagnosis, prognosis, and therapeutic decision making

24 Cf. Isabelle Stengers, *The Invention of Modern Science,* trans. Daniel Smith (Minneapolis: University of Minnesota Press, 2000).

are all supported by a succession of clinical and experimental studies and laboratory tests, in the course of which patients are treated not like subjects of their disease, but like objects.[25]

Initially, the "thingification" Canguilhem raises here appears to be some sort of unwanted side effect of an almost indisputably effective epistemology. In fact, in lieu of speaking of the "thingification" of human subjects, with the term's patently pejorative connotations, a more neutral characterization no doubt could apply: patients are no longer, strictly speaking, the veritable objects of medicine.[26] For the methods – and attendant material – that enable the production of generalizable facts also lead to a greater distance of doctor from patient. These methods require less direct contact between the two, and so this distance is purely technical at first. The distance grew in the second half of the 19th century with the introduction of precision instruments such as stethoscopes and thermometers. It stretched further with blood and urine tests, microscopy, and the clinical–pathological conference, which established systematic correlations between the symptoms presented by a sick person during their lifetime and the results of pathology or autopsy. The clinical–pathological conference "underscored the ultimate meaningfulness of discrete disease entities and the social centrality of their diagnosis by focusing on the connection between clinical signs during life and postmortem appearances."[27] From the 1920s onwards, it gained further depth with the advent of instruments for measuring blood pressure, electrocardiograms and electroencephalograms, radiography, then pH measure-

25 Canguilhem, *Writings on Medicine,* 35.
26 The television drama *House* offers an illustration of this approach taken to its limit.
27 Rosenberg, *Our Present Complaint,* 18.

ments, blood counts, and ultimately genetic testing. This suite of techniques simply reinforced the separation of patient from disease, a separation lucidly analyzed by Canguilhem and today seemingly self-evident, reproduced anew in case after case. Indeed, these diagnostic methods and techniques are founded on the hypothesis that the bodily fragment, biopsy, urine sample, blood drawing, or visualization of internal organs make disease detectable independently of a given organism while representing this organism at the same time. "The medical act's scientificity [*scientificité*] bursts forth with the symbolic substitution of the laboratory exam for the consulting room. Meanwhile, the scale of the representational plane of pathological phenomena shifts, from the organ to the cell, the cell to the molecule,"[28] and then, the molecule to the gene.

Second Site: Diagnosis, a "Dating" Gesture.

Ever smaller entities refer to disease or draw attention to it via their specific states or configuration. They are, however, only in a position to represent an organism in its totality because a mechanistic understanding of disease took shape alongside diagnostic methods derived from these same entities. This also shapes expectations of diagnostic speech from within this medical logic: diagnosis becomes an exercise in dating, in marking a patient's arrival within the timeline of the natural history of a given disease.

In premodern times, disease identification relied on the individuated presentation of symptoms that therefore remained inaccessible and unreliable. "Diseases were seen as points in time, transient moments during a process that could follow anyone on a variety of possible

---

28 Georges Canguilhem, *Études d'histoire et de philosophie des sciences concernant les vivants et la vie* (Paris: Vrin, 2002), 418. Translation mine.

trajectories."[29] Towards the end of the 19th century, diseases had become well-defined entities in two respects: the relatively thorough identification of their underlying mechanisms and the determination of their clinical course. This way of seeing took shape in relation to the medical establishment's growing interest in infectious diseases. Thanks to bacteriological advances, notably those of Louis Pasteur in France and Robert Koch in Germany, medicine began to effectively counter the functional mechanisms of this kind of disease.

> Perhaps more fundamentally, germ theories constituted a powerful argument for a reductionist, mechanism-oriented way of thinking about the body and its felt malfunctions. These theories communicated metaphorically the notion of disease entity as an ideal type, abstracted from its particular manifestations.[30]

Soon this conception came to be a model for other kinds of disease. For every disease described well from a nosological point of view there corresponded a "natural history that – from both the physician's and the patient's perspective – formed a narrative."[31] Accordingly, the ideal diagnostic act consisted in dividing the patient up into parts with which to then situate her in relation to the more or less settled chronology of a particular disease or, as it were, in relation to its *natural history*.

This evolution can also be interpreted as a shift in diagnostic attention from symptoms to discrete signs:

> The invention of the stethoscope and its use in auscultation as codified in [Laënnac's] *De l'auscultation* mediate of 1819 led to the eclipse of the symptom by the

---

29 Rosenberg, *Our Present Complaint*, 18.
30 Ibid., 19.
31 Ibid.

sign. A symptom is something presented or offered by the patient; a sign, on the other hand, is something sought and obtained with the aid of medical instruments. The patient, as the bearer and frequent commentator of symptoms, was "placed in parentheses." A sign could sometimes reveal an illness before a symptom led to its being suspected.[32]

This early form of predictive diagnostic reconnaissance throws into sharp relief the changes that transpired within the patient as a person: as an individual, as a person suffering from an illness, the patient's importance is on the wane, at least when it comes to the construction of medical knowledge and its epistemological status. This trend increases when considering the discovery of typhus at the turn of the 20th century and with it a new kind of patient – the otherwise healthy disease carrier. This notion came to have still greater bearing through genetics. Effectively, people of this kind appear to be like time bombs, whether for themselves and their loved ones or for their progeny, like "infected individuals without symptoms, 'hidden' vectors that must be detected."[33] In such light, the object of preventative hygiene is no longer the individual but a population requiring statistical management. Hence, in the name of focusing on the disease itself along with preventative hygiene, "placing the patient in parentheses," to take up Canguilhem's terms, is one of the conditions of possibility for the existence of modern, scientific medicine.

Consequently, within this regime of knowledge, a disease state can be diagnosed and described if and only if it obeys a causal and mechanistic logic, irrespective of

---

32 Georges Canguilhem, *A Vital Rationalist: Selected Writings from Georges Canguilhem*, ed. François Delaporte, trans. Arthur Goldhammer (New York: Zone Books, 1993), 141. Translation modified.

33 Jean-Paul Gaudillière, *La médecine et les sciences. XIXe et XXe siècles* (Paris: La Découverte, 2006), 44. Translation mine.

whether it is already manifest in the form of discrete symptoms or signs. Disease states that fail to conform to such a logic are deemed "imaginary" or "psychosomatic" (a term in use since the 1930s) and referred on to psychology. Equally troubling are diseases that have been detected and explained without any therapeutic treatment in existence "yet"; so too are those conditions having advanced to a terminal stage meaning that the sick person is also dying. Such conditions ought to force medicine to reckon with its own limits. All too often, however, such diagnoses do not prevent the staging of extensive, demanding yet ultimately pointless attempts at treatment. Already in 1873, Littré and Robin's *Dictionnaire de medicine* warned against needless aggravations of patient suffering. The entry for "cacothanasia" (more commonly referred to today as "therapeutic obstinacy") reads: "A tendency among some physicians to exhaust all pharmaceutical means, up to and including the most intensive of these, and even in the absence of the slightest probability of saving the patient, thereby bringing torment upon them in their final moments and making their death more difficult."[34] In such circumstances, the struggle against disease, understood to be carefully separated from the patient, risks turning into a struggle *against* rather than *for* the sick person.

With the development of new therapeutic frameworks in the first half of the 20th century came further institutionalization of the imperative of scientific neutrality. At this time, the "double blind study" became the norm for the clinical phase of pharmacological studies. This new approach worked in tandem with efforts to conscript most if not all sick people into cohorts in the service of clinical experimentation. If the double blind study marks

34 Émile Littré and Charles Robin, *Dictionnaire de médicine de chirurgie, de pharmacie, de l'art vétérinaire et des sciences qui s'y rapportent,* 13th edn. (Paris: J.B. Baillière et fils, 1873). Translation mine.

the zenith of the separation of sick person and disease, it also dramatically heralds a parallel phenomenon, which Canguilhem calls the interruption of dialogue between patient and physician. For "under this model of maximum control and outsourced judgment, physicians would see patients but ceased making decisions about particular treatment options and their sequencing, or even the analysis of their effects."[35]

Medical rationality, as Canguilhem remarks, only achieves its highest form when it manages to recognize its own limits, which should be "understood not as the failure of an ambition having proven its legitimacy time and again but rather as an obligation to shift register. [...] It must be conceded that the sick person is more than and different from a grammatical subject qualified by some attribute taken from the going nosology."[36] Canguilhem here issues a warning against the would-be unbridled rationalization of medical practice within which he detects a decisive aspect of the "claim to individual autonomy regarding health's appreciation and handling."[37] Up to this point, I find Canguilhem's claims to be compelling. I demur, however, when he submits that such conclusions make him fear a "revival of pre-rational forms of medicine."[38] Such misgivings, it seems to me, are symptomatic of an epistemology claiming to be the "rearguard"[39] of scientific knowledge processes: the one following in the other's footsteps, it risks making the same mistakes. Hence the persistent suspicion towards any and all practices that successfully treat disease by means other than those of Western allopathic medicine, whether in terms

35 Gaudillière, *La médecine et les sciences*, 90. Translation mine.
36 Canguilhem, *Études d'histoire et de philosophie des sciences*, 408–9. Translation mine.
37 Ibid, 404. Translation mine.
38 Ibid. Translation mine.
39 François Bing and Jean-François Braunstein, "Entretien avec Georges Canguilhem," *Interdisciplines* 1 (1984): 21–34.

of *curing* disease or *caring for* a person's relationship with disease. It is as if medicine becomes scientific "at long last" – in aiming to define itself in opposition to forms of medicine thereby deemed "premodern" and in permanently escaping charges of irrationality. In so doing, however, it finds it has no choice but to integrate its arch nemesis into its own methods, turning it into a specter that haunts medicine to this day. As the next section shows, the separation of disease and sick person and the attendant interruption of meaningful dialogue between doctor and patient culminate in the procedures underlying clinical and pharmaceutical double-blind studies. When viewed from this new perspective, it turns out that the fulcrum of these practices is forged from a morbid fear of irrationality and, more specifically, from the terror of being duped.

This threat is made flesh in the disobedient and irrational bodies of patients on the one hand, and in the unscientific healers henceforth relegated to the ranks of quackery on the other. Overcoming this threat calls for sophisticated defensive spells with the ability to defeat (as conclusively as possible) these enemies who continue to make life difficult for medicine. Such a defeat would turn medicine into the universal bearer of credible expert knowledge of disease. However, borne upon the terror of being duped and the will to dominate knowledge, this defensive spell comes at a price: the a priori dismissal of a whole range of practices, no matter their former, current, or possible effectiveness.

Third Site: Disqualifications

> *One thing is clear to me these days, there is a sinister inductive
> relationship between a fatal diagnosis being revealed and its
> being fulfilled, especially when it comes to so-called incurable
> diseases. [...] I was lucky enough, soon after taking in poisonous
> words, to get antidote words. They came from a realm beyond
> my own upbringing, from the mouth of renowned Fula healer
> Thierno Sadou Baa [...]: 'Where I come from, in Africa, this bad
> thing has already been in existence for a long time; some live
> their whole lives with it whereas others die from it quickly. White
> people have only just discovered this invisible thing with their
> instruments and this vision's revelation will kill more people
> than the bad thing itself, from the fear that it unleashes.'*
> – Julie[40]

The modern sciences created their own evidentiary criteria. Indeed, what characterizes the trustworthiness of
their material witnesses is that no sooner have they acquired the status of knowledge objects than they take on
an autonomous and atemporal mode of existence, one
independent of their creators along with the circumstances of their making. The laws of motion, of atomic
physics, and more recently entities like the neutrino or
DNA are examples of this kind of experimental achieve-
ment, which Isabelle Stengers contends is "the invention
of the power to confer on things the power of conferring
on the experimenter the power to speak in their name."[41]

I have already alluded to Galileo's experiment with the
inclined plane, a crucial experiment that would lead to
a formulation of the laws of motion. A closer examination of this experiment will help draw attention to the

40 Julie, writing on Dingdingdong's website, discusses testing "positive" for HIV in the 1980s: Julie, *Dingdingdong*, July 9, 2013, https://
dingdingdong.org/temoignages/julie/.
41 Stengers, *The Invention of the Modern Sciences*, 88.

difficulties that arise when transposing the experimental ideals of physics onto the life sciences, especially when it comes to the notion of the pathological. Like all modern experimental setups (and functioning to this day as the model thereof), Galileo's was highly artificial. In effect, the task was not to observe a falling body but to create a situation through which to make a judgment about how to characterize the motion of a body's fall: a perfectly smooth inclined plane upon which well-polished balls would roll (friction had to be at a minimum). This apparatus made it possible to vary the ball's descent. It transformed falling as a "natural" motion into a controllable phenomenon, which allowed it to be actively interrogated.

What Galileo thereby invented was the first

> *experimental apparatus,* in the modern sense of the term, an apparatus of which [he] is the *author,* in the strong sense of the term, as it consists of an artificial, premeditated setup that produces "facts of art" – artifacts in the positive sense. The singularity of this apparatus [...] *is that it allows its author to withdraw,* to let the motion testify in his place.[42]

Hence, once the variables are set (e.g., the ball's point of departure, the slope of the plane, etc.), Galileo *withdraws.* He lets the ball's motion answer all of the questions. It's up to nature to do what's left of the experimental work *all by itself.* What is conferred upon the experimental system, therefore, is the power of producing a fact of which the experimenter will subsequently attempt to convince her colleagues. According to such an approach, scientific facts are conceived of as neutral, universal, and independent of all opinions or personal interpretation. Because by withdrawing and making herself transparent in this way,

42 Ibid, 83. Translation modified.

the experimenter proves that not only is her experiment a success but, what's more, this success itself is in no way contingent upon her.

This kind of experimental neutrality, it should be noted, is not incompatible with the high degree of artifice within all experimental systems and the facts they produce. It is even more important not to conflate the implications of such artificiality – that facts are made or constructed – with the relativist position whereby facts are *merely* constructed. To the contrary, it is precisely because they are special *arte-facts*, ambitious in technical and historical terms, that they should not be considered less true or effective but rather hypereffective, in the sense of *having efficacy*. Events that bring "a new being or new method of measurement into existence"[43] deserve to be held in high regard if not celebrated, following Stengers, as products of a new kind of efficacy and a new kind of importance. But what would such a celebration look like? It might resemble what Bruno Latour calls the cult of *factishes* – a portmanteau of *fact* and *fetish*.[44] As Latour demonstrates, people who venerate fetishes harbor no illusions about the constructedness of their cult objects.

By introducing this neologism, Latour reminds us that, contrary to the Moderns' enlightened assumptions, practitioners of systems of so-called superstitious beliefs, for whom fetish worship plays a crucial role, are by no means dupes with respect to the constructedness of their cult objects. On the contrary, they are highly aware of the regulations that underlie the making of such objects, regulations that they follow and transmit. It is in this sense that we could learn from them, because they could teach us how to orient to celebrating well-made

---

43 Stengers, *Cosmopolitics I*, 32.

44 Bruno Latour, *On the Modern Cult of the Factish Gods*, trans. Heather MacLean and Catherine Porter (Durham: Duke University Press, 2010).

artifacts without discrediting them. The successful production of scientific facts might therefore be the centerpiece of a cult (read: culturing [*mise en culture*]) that
honors successful (read: efficacious) scientific artifacts.
At the same time, such a cult would be tasked with heeding the ways in which these facts are situated in context,
and thus with heeding their limits. The by-product of
artful experimenting, this cult would broach constructed
facts with breezy detachment but hold them in the highest regard. In the process, it could become a promising
defense mechanism against the universalizing claims of
the modern scientific attitude, in other words, against
the idea that facts produced in such and such a context
are correct and therefore automatically relevant to any
and all cases. Because this move, which accompanies the
so-called Modern attitude, amounts to discrediting all
practices that do not fit this mold. It is about celebration
without denunciation, celebrating the concrete existence
of the novel artifact as a world-changing force without
denouncing all others in return.

Such a cult would prevent us from forgetting that no
fact enjoys an autonomous existence: each and every fact
requires careful attention to endure and to find its true
value in the practical relations people maintain with it,
and not in the way these fall away. Hence, scientific facts
or factishes have an unstable mode of existence not unlike that of the *pharmakon,* the Greek term concurrently
referring to a poison, illicit substance, and medication.
Depending on the state the person receiving it is in, on
her environment but also the dosage she receives, a pharmakon can be toxic or therapeutic. Similarly, the transformative force of an artifact constitutively depends
upon its ability, within a particular milieu, to contribute
an active, compatible, and pertinent feature. This is why
the factish cult should also additionally and simultaneously be a cult of the *pharmakon,* a cult pursuing the task
of valuing the sophisticated and situated culture of sci-

entific practice, with all its accompanying requirements and obligations, without in the process elevating these to the status of universal norms.

When a practice loses sight of the situated existence of its productions and positions itself as sole bearer of knowledge about the "true" nature of the *pharmakon,* it inevitably becomes "incapable of what it is asking for, that is, a culture of usages."[45] This kind of culture is always situated and relational, as it demands a high degree of technical sophistication – the result of collective experimentation and development. That having been said, the judgment criteria for a usage practice or, put differently, evaluations of what it renders possible, cannot be determined a priori but only in the future anterior: "it will have been possible." The specifically Western problem that accordingly emerges is not, in the strict sense, the intrinsic instability of the *pharmakon,* its constitutive permanent openness, but rather the dread that this polysemy brings into being. The distinctiveness of this tradition inheres in its

> intolerance [...] towards this type of ambiguity, the dread it arouses. There has to be a fixed point, a foundation, or a guarantee. There has to be a stable distinction between helpful medication and harmful drug, between rational pedagogy and suggestive influence, between reason and opinion.[46]

As Stengers carefully demonstrates, the case of Anton Mesmer (1734–1815) is typical of the risk of denunciation and discrediting, a risk brought by medicine upon practices whose effects cannot be clearly ascribed. In 1784, Mesmer subjected his particular healing practice,

---

45 Tobie Nathan and Isabelle Stengers, *Doctors and Healers* (Oxford: Oxford University Press, 2018), 155. Translation modified.
46 Stengers, *Cosmopolitics I,* 29. Translation modified.

animal magnetism, to evaluation by the Académie Française. Having conducted a whole range of experiments, the committee tasked with passing judgment arrived at the following conclusion: "the fluid is powerless without imagination, while the imagination without the fluid is able to produce the effects that are attributed to the fluid"[47] Put simply, they proclaim that the fluid does not exist and turn Mesmer into a quack because his success, in their view, could only be credited to the imagination. The fluid, as it proved incapable of being transformed into a trustworthy witness, was deemed purely fictional and disqualified accordingly. To be sure, Mesmer did heal, in fact this was the finding their experiments produced. Evidently, however, he healed through fantastical means, with doubtful cause and effect relationships, and thus for the "wrong" reasons. There was no way of locating these "wrong" reasons. It was impossible to establish whether they took root in the healer's practices, in the patient's imagination, or in the relationship between the two.

We could tell a similar story from around the same time about Samuel Hahnemann (1755–1843), who tried to make room for homeopathy within the process of modern medicine's progressive establishment. From the outset, his principle that "like is cured by like" (*similia similibus curantur*) by way of almost imperceptibly low dosing – that he developed, what's more, through self-experimentation – went against the epistemological grain of unequivocal causal logic. Albeit for different reasons than in Mesmer's case, homeopathic healing practices also faced and continue to face repeated refusal from representatives of modern medicine. A German encyclopedia published in the 1880s carries an entry for homeopathy that reads as follows:

47 Nathan and Stengers, *Doctors and Healers*, 93.

We would need to go to great lengths to delineate this mystical system, which systematically contradicts the experiments of chemistry, physics, and pathology and which, in lieu of findings, is based entirely on unfounded beliefs. Moreover, it would be simply impossible to provide a faithful account of the many changes that homeopathy undergoes daily. [...] This sample should be enough to show that homeopathy places a greater burden on the healthy mind than on the sick body.

These two cases show how, from the outset, modern medicine based its identity on positing the refusal of the practices of "quacks" such as Mesmer, Hahnemann, and many others who healed for the "wrong" reasons. Alongside this sits a general opposition towards the body of the sick person, her living and suffering body. Patients themselves rarely coincide with preexisting categories. Hence when their conditions improve for reasons unaccounted for within a knowledge regime staked upon neutrality and objectivity, they are nothing other than the quack's accomplices. Whereas other sciences such as physics are constructed on the achievements of their practitioners, what makes modern medicine distinctive is its foundational frustration: frustration over the way living bodies tend to refuse to behave like reliable witnesses, namely unequivocally and consistently, and also frustration over the manner in which patients as well as physicians hold interests, ideas, and aspirations that risk uncontrollably overwhelming the therapeutic process.

The committee that evaluated animal magnetism advanced three reasons for explaining Mesmer's success despite the observed non-existence of the fluid: first, the healing powers of nature; second, the fact that Mesmer's patients stopped previously prescribed and highly toxic medication; third, the trust that patients placed in Mesmer's practice. The third reason is of particular interest to medical practice today, as it represents the driving

force behind the procedures leading up to formal recognition of a novel compound. Known as "the placebo
effect," the therapeutic power (*force*) of trust, hope, and
salutary faith constitutes an integral component of contemporary protocols surrounding decisions to authorize
the distribution of novel forms of medication. Current
medicine therefore officially recognizes these therapeutic effects, yet it does so in a negative mode. Indeed, the
double-blind study, where neither patient nor physician
know whether the treatment underway is the experimental medication (*verum*) or the placebo, is specifically
aimed at drawing a clear distinction between effects that
can be attributed to patients' beliefs or aspirations and
those due to the chemical compound itself. This triage
allows for the simultaneous conjuring and control of the
dangers of subjective influence that threaten the forward
progress of medicine. The strategy behind double-blind
studies therefore amounts to incorporating the enemy so
as to master it once and for all. The placebo effect is the
quack's counterpart, as it were, within modern medical
pharmacology.

Medical historian Philippe Pignarre has demonstrated
that the problematic nature of the placebo has little to do
with its methodological function as an innocuous compound deployed as a point of reference and comparison
in clinical studies for novel treatment options. Instead,
the method of the double-blind study became genuinely
troubling when it evolved from a technical and methodological reality into a political technique.[48] But what does

48 Pignarre's publications on medication are not yet available in English translation. Major texts include *Les deux médecines. Médicaments,
psychotropes et suggestion thérapeutique* (Paris: La Découverte, 1995); *Le
grand secret de l'industrie pharmaceutique* (Paris: La Découverte, 2003);
and, in collaboration with François Dagognet, *100 mots pour comprendre les medicaments. Comment on vous soigne* (Paris: Les Empêcheurs de
penser en rond, 2005). While not its central concern, some key aspects of Pignarre's critical theories on treatment and healing can be

he mean by this? The prevailing understanding of the placebo dates back to the early 19th century, yet despite this the wide-scale use of double-blind studies only took off in the 1970s. Within the pharmacological research community, it soon became clear that the placebo's presumed null effect was not absolute. In fact, it turned out that patients given a placebo tended to be in better health after the end of an experimental study than those given no treatment at all. Such findings inevitably raised the question of who was responsible for these "irrational" improvements. There was an easy answer: "We are – us doctors! It's our doing, it's our influence!" This answer turns the placebo effect into a political formula: not only does it *authorize* modern Western medicine's representatives to reevaluate the importance of their role in curing patients but it also *disqualifies* anew any way of practicing treatment otherwise and anyone who would do so. Moreover, the formula holds a new assumption: "You claim to hold secret knowledge allowing you to intervene upon the bodies of your patients. We can do exactly the same thing." Modern medicine therefore claims two powers for itself. It can heal in the same way traditional medicine heals and, *at the same time,* there is nothing secret or ambiguous about it thanks to scientific measurement. A duty falls upon modern medicine as a result of this capture: to "enlighten" gullible patients and warn them against all the quacks whose practices amount to nothing more or less than a repackaged placebo effect. Which brings us to posit the following questions:

If there are practitioners out there who know how to "maximize" the placebo effect, does it not deserve another name? It warrants consideration in terms that

found in a volume written with Isabelle Stengers: Philippe Pignarre and Isabelle Stengers, *Capitalist Sorcery: Breaking the Spell* (New York: Palgrave Macmillan, 2011).

don't disqualify it from the outset, does it not? It is up to us to strive to follow these practitioners and understand their practice in its specificity rather than dismissing it out of hand, is it not? Are there no cultures out there that have devised ways of sharing these techniques?[49]

Is it not the case that the risks that this disqualifying move brings on augur far graver consequences, at every level, than the risks that arise from plainly recognizing, as Canguilhem suggests, the "limits of medical rationality"? In truth, what is at stake is the disappearance of a whole range of practices. These practices know how to do a lot of things about which we still have so much to learn. Stemming from Western and non-Western traditions alike, they can be the stuff of inspiration precisely because, as Tobie Nathan explains, they "think things through against the medical grain, if you will, often taking disease to be a form of ordination, both the message and first move of a process of initiation into personhood."[50] A good place to start might be to learn how to constructively compose a life with a disease that modern medicine deems incurable and so puts off as a subject for future study. In putting things off to an indeterminate future horizon, what medicine displays is, above all, confusion over its own limits. It imagines these limits represent a passing phase when they are, in fact, an organizing principle. It goes something like this: "We do not *yet* know, we cannot *yet* heal this disease – but this will pass! It is just a matter of keeping calm and carrying on until a settled therapeutic treatment comes to market." To be sure, adopting a defensive attitude towards absent knowledge

---

49 Pignarre and Dagognet, *100 mots pour comprendre*, 250. Translation mine.

50 Tobie Nathan, *Psychothérapies* (Paris: Odile Jacob, 1998), 96. Translation mine.

helps drive and renew interest in medical research: the horizon beyond knowledge is a frontier awaiting conquest. From this perspective, however, we would overlook the fact that all new discoveries, no matter how revolutionary, inevitably conjure fresh knowledge remnants and yearnings. Medicine could take another path and, in addition to medical research, turn its attention to a time beyond the limit of its own horizons and remain open at the level of practice to collaborations and perspectives coming from other fields.

When it comes to the predictive diagnosis of incurable disease, bioethics may seem to be the most compelling direction at first. Yet I do not believe it is the most promising. Indeed, Niklas Luhmann makes a convincing argument when he writes that bioethics is a "sedative" and that society writes its own prescriptions "while moralists themselves have gone crazy."[51] Despite its best intentions, this sedative often clouds the "clear vision" we might have of new technologies and their dangers, and even tends to legitimate them, albeit in a roundabout way. Following Luhmann, German philosopher Petra Gehring writes: "far from destroying faith in technoscientific 'possibilities,' [bioethics] reaffirms it."[52]

Understanding why we need to take another direction entirely calls for something more than these few lines of criticism. In order to go a little further, I submit that two of bioethics' underlying assumptions merit questioning. Firstly, bioethics aims at "shedding light" (*éclairer*) on matters, which positions it within the Enlightenment tradition, consequently addressing itself to sovereign, conscious, autonomous subjects – in a word, solitary

---

51 Niklas Luhmann, *Die Wissenschaft der Gesellschaft* (Frankfurt am Main: Suhrkamp Verlag, 1990), 697. Translation mine.
52 Petra Gehring, "Fragliche Expertise. Zur Etablierung von Bioethik in Deutschland," in *Wissenschaft und Demokratie*, ed. Michael Hagner (Frankfurt-am-Mein: Suhrkamp Verlag, 2012), 112–39, at 134. Translation mine.

ones. It is precisely this inheritance that makes bioethics incapable of cultivating a situation from within, which is a practice that goes hand in hand with collective action. Secondly, because bioethics came about in response to technological innovation, it only tends to fulfill its role after the fact, as an agent for regulating and curtailing "collateral damage." In other words, bioethics is content to track down solutions for "ready-made" problems that others put before it. This kind of orientation explains why bioethics all too often lacks imagination, or rather, the ability to let itself imagine things otherwise. Hence, it belongs to an epistemological and institutional logic that prevents it from finding a way to construct its own problems rather than reacting to preexisting ones.

For these reasons, I believe that in order to begin building a more appropriate milieu – one more richly populated and ready to make our creature, the predictive test, welcome – it is worth turning our attention to horizons beyond bioethics. In this second chapter, we have traversed a range of historical and conceptual domains that provided greater purchase on some moments of bifurcation, moments when other things, paths, or practices might have been possible. By taking such stories in, we will have equipped ourselves with the means to begin spotting camels, that is to say, with the tools to begin constructing problem-solutions anew. Unfortunately, what is before us is not the *one* good camel that can solve things once and for all. Rather, it is the beginning of a collection of camels, who will need to be nourished, cared for, and tamed from within the very practices under cultivation.

In the third and final chapter, I will attempt an initial proposition for a more satisfactory construction of these problems. The perspectives discussed next are not in any way intended as recipes. I will not attempt to write up a new version of the "Guidelines for Molecular Genetics Predictive Test in Huntington's Disease." My propositions will have completed their journey once they manage to enrich the imagination of the actors who find themselves entangled in some manner or another in the predictive test for HD, or, to put things differently, once they manage to populate our creature's milieu with less moribund and terrifying and more hospitable beings.

3

Artisans of Becoming

"Speculative Narration"

> *Stories are much bigger than ideologies. In that is our hope.*
> – Donna Haraway[1]

When you search for "Huntington's disease" on YouTube, two kinds of results come up. The first are short films produced in the style of an infomercial: in the most dispassionate of tones, they explain HD by way of diagrams that indicate symptoms, clinical progression, and the care options available. The second type of content douses the viewer with countless private clips. For the most part, the production quality of these clips is basic and they bear all the hallmarks of the horror story. Picture a room, covered in dust: a frightfully thin woman appears, wanders about like a crazy person, her obvious distress is upsetting to behold, she flails about, falls, staggers and sways. Such footage is cut together with tales of people with early-onset or juvenile HD. You can watch adorable little kids, running all over the place and yet transforming, slowly, into invalids, agitated at first and then becoming listless, the whole thing accompanied by commentary shot

1 Donna J. Haraway, *The Companion Species Manifesto: Dogs, People and Significant Otherness* (Chicago: University of Chicago Press, 2003), 17.

through with fear and despair from scared parents, children, brothers, and sisters. The HD imagery and discourse circulated by medicine and the public turns the disease into a monstrous and inescapable form of current day possession, and it reaches new intensities in testimonials from the very people concerned by the disease, whether these testimonials are intended as pedagogy and explanation or whether they are simply direct manifestations of solitude and plight.

In October 2013, an altogether different kind of video joined this content: "A Message from Doctor Olivier Marboeuf."[2] It is a video monologue given by a neurologist in which he recounts the founding of an experimental, multidisciplinary research unit dedicated to HD and its associated tests, conceived collectively by those giving as well as receiving care. Doctor Marboeuf begins his tale by relating how, in light of the position he holds within a French center offering predictive testing, he often finds himself having to announce test results to at-risk persons. He sits throughout the video in his practice, behind his desk. Evidently, he is addressing an audience of his medical "peers" on the one hand and, on the other, people who are concerned with the sickness in some way: at-risk persons, family members, or caregivers.

He explains that he wants to relate his encounter with a patient and her sister along with the effect this meeting had on him. One year earlier, these two women had set a challenge for him that he had never faced before: to call his own practice into question along with everything he believed he knew about Huntington's disease itself, its symptoms, its tragic nature, and its clinical progression. It all started when he confronted the young woman with the revelation of her unfavorable genetic status,

2   Unité Expérimentale Alice Rivières, "#1 Dr Marboeuf sur la maladie de Huntington (Huntington's disease)," *YouTube*, October 21, 2013, https://youtu.be/S1WqbRB9a6Q.

first announcing her CAG count, then going on to provide her with the usual information about the psychological, medical, and social assistance she could receive. This patient reacted in a way that no other patient had before: she burst into rage. In terms both harsh and to the point, she told him that never again under any circumstances did she wish to be in contact with him or anyone from his team, nor did she wish to take up their offers of assistance. And then she left, slamming the door behind her, leaving him utterly thrown.

A few months later, Doctor Marboeuf explains, this patient's sister called him and scheduled an appointment. The two women turned up together, but it was the sister who led the discussion. She too gave him explicit criticism, taking him on time and again: "How do you know what will happen to my sister?" "How do you know *exactly* what will happen to my sister *in particular*?" He relates how he tried to justify himself, by replying that it was his duty as a specialist to inform patients with precision, to be clear, to not raise false hopes and so on and so forth. The sister shot back: "but why don't you say that *you don't know*?" It would not be appropriate given his role as a physician, he said. She pressed the point: "There are people who say that *they don't know*." This is what happens, she went on to explain, in the Dutch city of Apeldoorn at the Atlant Center. She went for a visit and the treatment options she observed were, in her view, nothing short of amazing. People with Huntington's in residence at the center were in no ways in a pitiful state despite the advanced nature of their condition. They seemed to be living happily. When, at the end of the conversation, he bid adieu to the two women with an "I hope to see you soon," the sister plainly laid down their terms: "We will only come back once you are able to tell us that *you don't know*." Frustrated, and a little irritated, he let them go, saying it was unlikely the day would come when he would see them again.

He goes on to explain in the video that these encounters nonetheless piqued his curiosity. In June of 2013, he made the most of a conference in the Netherlands to stay an extra day and pay a visit to Apeldoorn and the Atlant Center. "I have to admit, it is impressive," he concedes. Patients' day-to-day lives and care were organized, he noted, in a tailored fashion. Upon returning to France, Doctor Marboeuf wondered what he could do. To be sure, given what he had experienced at the Atlant Center, the demands his patient and her sister had made seemed distinctly less egregious. The sister, he has to admit, "is not wrong." At this point – and with this his creation story draws to a close – he decides to take a proposal to his managers, to initiate a small experimental research unit dedicated to various aspects of Huntington's disease and its test, a co-construction to be undertaken in concert with patients and their families. In September 2013, management authorized the creation of the unit bearing the name of Alice Rivières. Since March 2014, patients and their families have been working together with caregivers and doctors and, as Doctor Marboeuf announces at the end, this is just the beginning!

Where the closing credits would role, a single sentence flashes up: "Communication posted on YouTube on the 17th of September 2014, from a possible world to be built together." This sentence alone reveals that the film is not a documentary but a fabulation. First of all, because of the date stamp: the video was initially presented in the context of a world congress on Huntington's disease held in September 2013 in Rio de Janeiro before being uploaded to YouTube. Doctor Marboeuf's story would have had to unfold in the future. And if you search a little harder, you will find no sign of the Alice Rivières Unit other than this video. Is it therefore a hoax? No, it's a lure!

This film is the outcome of a collaboration between filmmaker and Dingdingdong member Fabrizio Terranova and storyteller-cum-performance artist Olivier

Marboeuf. As I have in this book, these two artists took Alice Rivières's story as their starting point, relaying it in their own way, in keeping with the operating principle that drives Dingdingdong, a collective dedicated to coproducing knowledge about Huntington's. This principle holds that we actually must "lather" the ideas that animate us, taking them up again over time from various perspectives and thus lending them consistency, a thickness of their own. I have no doubt that this work of taking and retaking, of successive acts of giving form (*mise en forme*) is needed to arrive at the point where concepts are sufficiently specified and, thereby and thereupon, made to become ever more real. While Alice's story put an obligation before me – to dive into the histories of predictive testing and modern medicine the better to understand their stakes – for Terranova and Marboeuf it presented an opportunity to cultivate a new kind of narrative: "speculative narration." The ways of doing and the strategies that this narration deploys aim, quite literally, "to gather together the conditions of possibility for making an idea, one for which there can be no guarantees, become true."[3] This is not intended in a general sense but rather in relation to concrete and specific situations of conflict and powerlessness. Speculative narration therefore intends to contrast "predetermined" paths with stories of how things could be otherwise; the latter rub the former against the grain and influence them.[4] Unlike what usually happens in science fiction, the story Mar-

3 Thierry Drumm, personal communication, 2014.
4 This approach is altogether different from so-called "narrative ethics." Narrative ethics derives ethical or moral maxims from the analysis of more or less canonical literary texts. Here, the filmmakers explicitly conceive of their video as a form of ethical and political engagement within the field of presymptomatic diagnosis itself. Moreover, they take up "speculative narration" beyond this particular context and are, especially in the case of Fabrizio Terranova, committed to developing this form of practice. See Didier Debaise et al., "Speculative Narration: A Conversation with Valérie Pihet, Di-

boeuf recounts does not take place in a faraway future, whether in temporal or situational terms. Rather, it takes a real situation as its starting point and spins, threads, or weaves it by introducing slight adjustments and prudent additions that, although minor, prove decisive. Hence, no gulf separates historical reality from storytelling reality. Nothing improbable or impossible happens. The point is neither to sketch out a *utopia* (a non-place) or a *uchronia* (a non-time), nor to conduct a thought experiment extrapolating upon the effects of various counterfactuals.

Instead, Olivier Marboeuf (the storyteller), a.k.a. Doctor Marboeuf (the narrator), *fabulates* a situation for the camera based on a future soon to come. In this situation, a number of true-to-life elements – the anger of test subjects, notions of the right to know and not to know, experiences gleaned from Apeldoorn's Atlant Center – conspire to lay the groundwork for the possibility of creating a research laboratory with the task of inaugurating and investigating new versions of Huntington's disease. His story foretells every step of the journey needed to achieve this kind of encounter. The strategy he adopts, therefore, is one of narrative awareness raising. Although fashioned from the future, it remains faithful to known, situated, and contested reality. At the same time, by way of an equally situated and effective process of thinking through, this story strives to make the disease and testing for it awaken to another life.

To be sure, the narrator constructed his account from elements that were "given" to him. Olivier Marboeuf did not know about HD before undertaking this work and drew on to what we told him. However, by taking this as a basis for improvisation, he managed to reconfigure these elements on his own terms and produce an original story with the power to surprise his tutors and give their

dier Debaise, Katrin Solhdju, and Fabrizio Terranova," *Parse* 7 (2017): 65–77.

thinking new purchase. A noteworthy example is the crucial proposition that the sister intervene and specifically demand that the doctor must recognize he cannot know what will happen to his patient. This demand constitutes the piece's narrative center and can be understood in three different ways.

Firstly, it is the expression of a refusal to become the passive victim of medical knowledge held up as absolute truth. Doctor Marboeuf must not act as if the predictive knowledge he is conveying amounts to the "definitive answer to a question posed once and for all." Instead, the sister makes a demand that forces Doctor Marboeuf to treat his announcement like an "indeterminate answer to a question prompted and created by a provisional desire to know,"[5] an answer providing a direction, yet which should in no way be taken as an exclusive explanation.

On another level, the sister pushes Doctor Marboeuf to support the idea that HD's course varies from one person to the next. A fortiori, she enjoins him not to confuse objective knowledge about a condition with the subjective experience of living with this condition. The distinction the English language draws (and the French does not) between the concepts of "disease" and "illness" makes this crucial difference plain to see. Whereas "disease" designates sickness as a medically defined entity and this "by contrast with other diseases," the concept of "illness" refers to the concrete and personal perspective of the sick person, to "what patients live through and describe." While sickness as "disease" is the ready object of medical diagnosis, "illness" evokes "the subjective feeling of lack of health that a person holds."[6] Taking stock

---

5 Paul-Loup Weil-Dubuc, "Les servitudes du droit de savoir: Autour du diagnostic présymptomatique," *La Vie des Idées*, 15 October 2013, http://www.laviedesidees.fr/les-servitudes-du-droit-de-savoir. html. Translation mine.

6 Henrike Hölzer, "Die Simulation von Arzt-Patienten-Kontakten in der medizinischen Ausbildung," in *Szenen des Erstkontakts zwischen*

of this distinction (and hence the multiple meanings or plural character of all disease) means coming to terms with some changes. A first consequence is the need to adopt a perspective whereby it becomes possible to take seriously and accompany patients as they suffer from symptoms even in the absence of a recognized, objective, or causally scripted condition in the sense of a "disease" (for example, some forms of chronic pain).[7] Moreover, the disease/illness distinction makes it possible to conceive of and even to conjure situations in which the disease is lived through in less dramatic terms than those predicted by diagnosis or prognosis. In fact, calls to systematically distinguish illness from disease, particularly within the field of nursing and care studies, are often motivated less out of ontological than pragmatist concerns where the aim is to produce concrete effects.[8] Giving full weight to this distinction makes it possible to put all relevant actors in a position to collectively compose diverse kinds of know-how about their sickness, know-how that need not privilege medical or scientific knowledge. According to this logic, patients (from the Latin "to suffer" or "to put up with") no longer have to passively endure the disease whose active "management" is the sole preserve of medicine. They can instead take up an expert role when it comes to at least one fundamental aspect: how illness is experienced and what its usages are in their everyday life, a form of knowledge that they alone can convey. Such a perspective is paramount: it is a prerequisite to any co-

---

Arzt und Patient, eds. Walter Bruchhausen and Céline Kaiser (Bonn: Bonn University Press, 2012), 107–17, at 112. Translation mine.

7   Regarding "medically unexplained symptoms," see Monica Greco, "The Classification and Nomenclature of 'Medically Unexplained Symptoms': Conflict, Performativity and Critique," *Social Science & Medicine* 75 (2012): 2362–69.

8   Here, "pragmatism" is to be understood in William James's sense of the word.

construction of knowledge about Huntington's and other conditions.

> The well-known slogan, "My womb belongs to me," could certainly be discussed for its simplicity and individualism. But if we understand what started the women moving, it was move like "My womb does not belong to you," and there any individualist simplification disappears. It is a real "hands off!" shouted at all those who, in the interests of the state or of morality, want to charge of women's wombs.[9]

In the same way, thinking with the distinction between "disease" and "illness," we can hear a nuance in the demand made upon Doctor Marboeuf: "at least admit that the truth of our disease does not belong to you or, at any rate, not only to you."

There is a third reading of this demand. It can be understood as a way of standing the much-debated at-risk person's right not to know on its head. This right, when it comes to Huntington's disease, is conveyed in the *Guidelines* discussed earlier through the explicit recommendation not to undertake prenatal testing for HD unless the parents are sure they will terminate the pregnancy should the embryo test positive. This would otherwise amount to depriving the child brought into the world of the right not to know, for she would be born in the knowledge she was a gene-carrier rather than an at-risk person. In narratively assembling an inversion of this right together with his patient's rage, Marboeuf fabulates an interesting version of the doctor's duty to not only be aware of the limits to his own knowledge but also to expressly convey these to his patients. He will only become worthy of his patients when he is ready to heed this twofold duty.

9   Tobie Nathan and Isabelle Stengers, *Doctors and Healers* (Oxford: Oxford University Press, 2018), 151.

One of the strengths of Marboeuf's monologue lies in that he seizes upon what is at stake in our exploration. He does so by refraining from presenting the doctor's re-orientation as a sudden conversion, instead dramatizing it as an arduous and protracted process. Indeed, as he tells it, Doctor Marboeuf approaches the demand that he say, "I don't know," with the skepticism of a medical professional. For this requirement runs against his de-ontological allegiances. He insists that he must inform. For him, this is a professional duty. He thus reminds us of the existence of a conflict, one in which doctors often find themselves embroiled, "conflicts of interest between, for example, the individual physician's duties to a patient and his loyalty to the profession, as when his conduct is criticized as 'unprofessional' for harming, not his clients, but rather his colleagues."[10] Marboeuf's story therefore draws its speculative power specifically from the fact that it does not wantonly dismiss the duties felt by the doctor towards the medical profession, duties that make sense to him and guide his practice – duties that he would neglect were he to be overcome with compassion or were he to say or even just whisper the words, "I don't know." A new possibility can only emerge when Doctor Marboeuf allows the sister's provocation, which leaves him bereft at first ("We will only come back when you are ready to say, 'I don't know'"), to resonate and give him pause. In the end, we cannot know whether or not he says, "I don't know." What is truly significant, however, is the narrative shift that resulted in his appropriating this injunction and giving it the authority to become his vocation, his calling. He dedicated the time and effort needed to a project that allowed him to transform this provocation, little by little, into the cornerstone of a research laboratory organized in a truly coproductive manner. From within

10 Stephen Toulmin, "How Medicine Saved the Life of Ethics," *Perspectives in Biology and Medicine* 25, no. 4 (1982): 736–50.

the hospital milieu itself and together with representatives from all involved parties, he decided to examine the merits of the professional, familial, and moral duties and demands felt by one and all, along with their reciprocal influences. In short, the research unit that Marboeuf fabulates on the basis of a possible world to be built together is one based on the experience that a person might need to place themselves in jeopardy (*se compromettre*), to let go of "what they hold dear,"[11] if what counts is *becoming respons-able*, that is becoming capable of answering for one's own practice and its objects.[12]

Rewriting Natural History

> *The moral or political concern running through pragmatism is precisely to preserve, as much as can be, the subject's ability to act, her confidence in a possible action in the world.*
> — Didier Debaise[13]

At first, it seems curious that this fabulation should choose the very caregivers of an establishment dedicated to Huntington's to say the line "we do not know." After all, it would seem reasonable to assume that the experienced personnel working there would have a particularly keen and thoroughgoing understanding of what happens after presymptomatic testing and particularly regarding the initial onset of symptoms. When it comes to the collective task of apprehending HD differently, the very crux of the Dingdingdong project, everyone brings their own

---

11 Émilie Hache, *Ce à quoi nous tenons* (Paris: La Découverte, 2011).

12 For a discussion of the notion of "response-ability," see Donna J. Haraway, *When Species Meet* (Minneapolis: University of Minnesota Press, 2008).

13 Didier Debaise, "La pensée laboratoire: Une approche pragmatique de la connaissance," in *Éduquer dans le monde contemporain: Les savoirs et la société de la connaissance,* eds. Ali Benmakhlouf and Nicolas Piqué (Casablanca: Le Fennec, 2013), 63–74, at 69.

ways of pursuing an inquiry and conveying it. Hence, such inquiries are often communal. They are something of a spring into which no one ever wades alone because each of us is always connected to the rest of the group, even if only to fuel our appetites with fresh data and experiences, putting them to collective work. Accordingly, Marboeuf's video drew in particular on two field-work trips to Apeldoorn along with the discussions and interactions we had with personnel and patients there. If Apeldoorn seemed like "paradise for Huntington's" to us, it was not because the disease became something pleasant there. Rather, it was because the care this place achieved, through perpetual coproduction with sick people and their kin, was remarkable for always tending toward the general wellbeing of those known there as "residents" rather than toward the management of "patients" and their symptoms.

At Apeldoorn, they cultivate the art of caring, an art whose theory and practice is made to measure. From our two visits, we were able to glean some aspects of this art that will, I hope, show how it is strategically accompanied by a form of "non-knowledge" about HD. Marboeuf the storyteller, following the lead of his patient's sister, finds among Apeldoorn's caregivers the ability to admit not knowing what will happen for such and such a gene carrier. In so doing, he translates a whole range of observations about the details of their practices, of clues and experimental ways of composing something from HD's puzzles that form the caregivers' very modus operandi. The fact remains that the manner in which people live with Huntington's at Apeldoorn brings about a less dramatic, tragic, and cruel version of the disease. At Heemhof, which is the Atlant Center's long-term assisted living center for Huntington's patients, everything is staked on ensuring that patients, who are admitted when their condition reaches a particularly advanced stage, have the opportunity to remain or become the creators or protago-nists of their own disease.[14]

In this chapter, I have decided to describe the obser-vations and discussions we had at Apeldoorn in some detail. This choice follows from my conviction that all caregiving situations play a decisive role in lending con-sistency to the milieu surrounding the test-creature, as much so as the epistemological and ethical prescriptions that structure the medical field. In any case, it is easy enough to imagine that a future with Huntington's is less terrifying if you foresee staying at a place like Heem-hof, rather than ending up, by default, in either a nurs-ing home, which is ill-equipped to deal with a condition that affects relatively young people, or an institution for people born with severe disability, which risks being just as inadequate. Unfortunately, to this day, in France and many other Western countries, these are by far the most common outcomes for HD patients (although the trend may be turning around thanks to the combined efforts of caregivers and patient associations).

The forms of support and care the Atlant Center pro-vides, which manage to make it possible to not only to live with the experience of HD but to live well with it, are the fruit of many years of experience. The center was founded some forty years ago, the Huntington's unit in 1992, and it continues to improve upon its practices, many of which were devised here. These practices have a range of temporalities. The relationship with a new "cli-ent" usually and preferably begins at a time when they are still in the early stages of being sick. In fact, quite of-ten at this time it is the loved ones who desire support, whereas the sick person often plainly refuses contact

14 Even though Apeldoorn serves here as a model, there are, of course other facilities (e.g., Hôpital Marin de Hendaye, in France) that tire-lessly develop and cultivate similarly rich approaches to patient-care.

with the medical services on offer. "Here, they perfectly understand that helping loved ones to help sick people provides the same amount of relief to both groups and helps to avoid many crises."[15]

The most active people during this phase are so-called "case managers."[16] They act as an interface between patients, families, and the institution itself. The nature of their work, in other words, is above all diplomatic. They keep in touch with the family, undertake home visits, and help loved ones prepare the sick person for the need to receive support. "There is always a solution to be found," says R., whose business card simply reads: *Case manager, Huntington*. R. operates on a case-by-case basis according to "a veritable casuistry: turning each case into an event."[17] To achieve this, she must use her imagination and find the tone and gestures suited for each situation. For instance, she recounted the case of a sick person who refused to have any contact whatsoever with her but whose family sought her help. As she knew he would regularly go into town for groceries, she decided she would cross paths with him one day as a way of making an initial contact. "There is always something you can help with, even if it's just something tiny. From there, you can build something." At first glance, this might seem to be quite an intrusive way of intervening, one that goes against the ethics of consent. Surely you shouldn't follow a sick person out getting groceries after they have refused to be in contact with you? If we take a closer look however,

15 Alice Rivières, "Apeldoorn 2012," *Dingdingdong*, December 5, 2012, https://dingdingdong.org/reportages/apeldoorn-2012. Translation mine.

16 This role has recently been introduced in France for people with Alzheimer's disease. A quite distinct version of this duty, known as the "coordinator for a program of care" (coordinateur de parcours de soin), is beginning to emerge for HD and other diseases whose oversight is particularly challenging.

17 Rivières, "Apeldoorn 2012."

what emerges is the careful and discrete construction of what anthropologists Antoine Hennion and Pierre Vidal-Naquet in their inquiry into home care refer to as a "situational ethics." Such an ethics achieves expression "within the course of acting itself. [...] To put it crudely, 'ethics is already within.' Actors are moral actors, even if they do not follow principles that can be articulated in a detached, general, or absolute fashion."[18] In effect, every situation of care is shot through with demands we would rather shy away from. It falls upon caregivers to guarantee the security and wellbeing of dependents and to respect their autonomy. At the same time, there is no escaping the fact that people receiving care regularly have to be made to do things they refuse to do or find pointless. Hence, in concrete practice, white lies, tricks, and workarounds frequently sustain the gestures and moves leading to a given goal.[19] Procedures such as these are *pragmatist* in the proper sense insofar as they characterize a practice whose effects are not measured against abstract principles: "not an unprincipled action, the justification for which changes randomly from one situation to the next, but an action whose principles are actualized in the course of its very enactment."[20]

In another stage in which the sick person, their loved ones, and staff from the Atlant Center come together, the

18 Antoine Hennion and Pierre A. Vidal-Naquet. "'Enfermer Maman!' Épreuves et arrangements: Le care comme éthique de situation," *Sciences sociales et santé* 33, no. 3 (2015): 65–90. See also Antoine Hennion et al., *Une ethnographie de la relation d'aide: de la ruse à la fiction, ou comment concilier protection et autonomie*, report for MiRe-DREES/CSI-Cerpe, 2012, http://hal-ensmp.archives-ouvertes.fr/hal-00722277.

19 Since the original publication of *Testing Knowledge*, Dingdingdong has achieved an inquiry that dives into the details of the incredible creativity invented by HD-patients, their families, and close ones. See Émilie Hermant and Valérie Pihet, *Le chemin des possibles. La maladie de Huntington au soin de ses usagers* (Paris: Éditions Dingdingdong, 2017).

20 Ibid.

sick person has agreed to work with caregivers but continues to live at home. At this point, their case manager works with them to craft a personalized program of home care, with both emotional and material components. Aside from help with washing, housework, and cooking, consideration is also given to occupational therapy, speech therapy, and psychiatric or psychological support. This is also the time when a discussion happens about equipment that will be useful but need to be ordered in: medical bed, walking frame, wheelchair, shower chair, etc. During this period, some choose to take up the offer of day care, another option Apeldoorn provides, with various support services and activities. This period is by no means conflict-free. R. must make sure to keep her practice fluid and open as order never lasts long. She has to pay constant attention to what is happening in order to spot and identify the slightest mishap and, as quickly as possible, conjure a corresponding proposition. Invariably, it is impossible to guarantee ahead of time that these propositions will succeed. They will prove their worth through their effects, as they are enacted as so many opportunities or "living hypotheses"[21] for better facing up to the situation at hand. If they fail, then another direction must be found. This thoughtful, pragmatist approach constantly makes do with uncertainties and, as it were, with non-knowledge.

In many cases, the question arises of whether a sick person is ready to move into Heemhof in order to receive care corresponding with their symptoms' progression and also to relieve their loved ones. Entering Heemhof, which is at a slight remove from the city of Apeldoorn itself, prompts immediate surprise. Nothing about the lighting, the smell, or the soundscape recalls the feelings

---

21 The expression is William James's, from *The Will to Believe and Other Essays in Popular Philosophy* (New York: Dover Publications, Inc., 1956), 2ff.

that tend to go with hospitals or support centers. Residents' individual rooms, kitchens, three large common rooms, entertainment areas, and various technical spaces open onto a square arrangement of wide corridors bathed in light. Residents can move about freely, they make their way through the corridors on foot or in electric wheelchairs, gaze into the distance, or smoke on the balconies appointed for this purpose. Each of them can arrange their room as they see fit, with their own furniture and selection of wall colors. It is even possible to keep small pets, provided the sick person or their family takes care of them – we made out rabbits, hamsters, and parakeets. We learn that there are as many caregivers working at Heemhof as there are patients in residence. If we take their working schedule into account, this means that during the day there is at least one caregiver for every three patients. Heemhof receives roughly three hundred Euros per patient per day in public funding; patients and their families make up the difference on an income-adjusted sliding scale.

Let us consider three aspects of the practices of living and caregiving that unfold at Heemhof: the color-coded system for collective crisis management, the use of *Video Interaction Guidance* (VIG)[22] and the multitude of objects invented to improve ordinary living. These techniques are elaborated as a veritable art of "listening, respecting, nourishing, and even enjoying [*jouir*] finite bodies."[23] M., one of the psychologists, explains the three-color system to us. Working closely with Heemhof's caregivers and case managers, he supports residents as well as home care patients and their families. In his view, the three-color system enables full time staff to collaborate

22 See the comprehensive website of the *British Association for Video Interaction Guidance UK,* https://www.videointeractionguidance.net/.
23 Annemarie Mol, *The Logic of Care: Health and the Problem of Patient Choice* (London: Routledge, 2008).

effectively with doctors, psychologists, and loved ones. Imagine a traffic sign: when everything is fine it shows green, hence green markings appear in the resident's file, updated daily. When small things start to go wrong and signs of frustration, anger, or impatience emerge the light turns orange. Red signals a full-blown crisis situation. The most important of the three colors is orange: it indicates the moment that calls for attention from the team and loved ones, forcing them to think in order to understand exactly what is happening and to agree on what needs to be put in place to avoid crisis if possible and turn things green again. Going on a walk, organizing a session with the psychologist, a trip to the city, a weekend at home – these different initiatives will each have to prove themselves against a situation bearing the mark of the notorious orange color. The three-color system therefore constantly accompanies loved ones and the multidisciplinary team, it allows and calls for careful, daily evaluation of each resident's situation and serves as an effective machine for collectively anticipating and averting crises.

Another form of crisis management is the regular use of VIG techniques. Dutch psychologist Harrie Biemans and his colleagues developed this method in the 1980s, which was then conceptually refined and extended by University of Edinburgh ethologist Colony Trevarthen. Biemans was interested, above all, in early interactions between parents and their children. He attempted to understand how dysfunction set in within this prelinguistic relationship and find ways of responding to it.

Since then, the method has gained traction primarily in England, the Netherlands, and Canada, each time in a version adapted to its local context of use: schools, hospitals, or workplace relations. Here is how it works: action sequences unfolding in a given setting (domestic or institutional) are first recorded and then prepared for viewing by someone referred to as a "guider." Then, most if not all the people involved in the sequence watch the footage with the guider and analyze it together. From the footage selection phase onwards, however, the focus is less on moments of crisis or failure than on moments of successful communication or interaction. Notably, the usage of video technology allows for the possibility of rewinding, for instance, from a relaxed scene in which mother and child are laughing together. By going back in time, it becomes possible to better understand and make explicit the steps leading up to this pleasant but potentially rare situation, the attitudes, gestures, or words that brought it about. By giving participants the means to take stock of the ways in which some of their interactions are successful, over time they become able to produce and stabilize some of their behaviors in situ, with a view to multiplying such felicitous moments.

At Apeldoorn, this method is put to two ends: first, to focus participants' attention on the times when their interactions succeed and, second, to turn the times when they experience serious difficulty into learning opportunities. If a given family laments repeated crises, a VIG-trained team is sent in to try and record one such situation. Then, the sick person along with the family, the team of caregivers, and the guider watch and discuss the video all together in order to understand what led to the crisis and what role each of them played in it. In such cases, the recordings become a source of inspiration the better to think through failed interactions with a given resident and to put in place strategies adapted to their needs. The process is repeated as many times as necessary. New caregivers also take part in these VIG sessions and train themselves through the collaborative screening and discussion. For privacy reasons, the videos are destroyed after analysis.

Finally, living with Huntington's at Heemhof is different in light of the material resources on hand. Residents have an impressive array of equipment at their disposal.

This allows them to keep up a surprisingly broad range of physical activities for as long as possible. Along with standing bicycles for going on walks with their loved ones and many other sophisticated devices (electric wheelchairs, walking aids, a variety of winches fitted to beds, showers, and baths), each sick person gets a "personal communicator." This is a "smart" touchscreen tablet with accessibility options allowing its continued use into the advanced stages of illness. If desired, the device accompanies Huntington's patients from the earliest stages and thus constitutes a kind of externalized memory. By way of a digital voice encoder, it enables them to continue to express themselves vocally and converse long after analog speech is no longer an option, using a sophisticated and effective system.[24] The team endeavors to convince residents to take up using this communication technology as well as electric wheelchairs as early as possible. Indeed, from their experience, the longer a person waits, the harder it is to learn these skills. If a person makes a few regular trips in an electric wheelchair while they can still walk, these skills are conserved much longer, even into the advanced stages of the disease. During our visits, we also encountered a resident at Heemhof who decided to undergo gastrostomy, that is to make use of a gastric tube to feed himself. Having serious difficulties with swallowing and suffocating – which are frequent issues at advanced stages and made each of his meals time-consuming, unpleasant, and nutritionally inadequate – this intervention allowed him to once again savor the tastes he most enjoyed. While he now feeds himself almost exclusively via gastric tube (for his caloric intake), he is free to eat and drink small quantities of the things that make him truly happy. In other words, he removed what amounted to obligatory force-feeding from his daily life

24 HD's motor symptoms lead to difficulties with the vocal apparatus, notably elocution and swallowing problems.

and, without it being systematically associated with the danger of "doing the wrong thing," he rediscovered the pleasure of enjoying his favorite meal: fries and a cold beer! In so doing, he teaches us that it is possible to situate this move not within a context of palliative care and its systematic association with "end of life" but instead within a context of living, plain and simple.

Alongside these high-tech tools, more mundane objects made on site play a vital role in everyday life. Consider the ashtrays. Wrought from salvaged materials, they are astounding creations. A metal ring is welded onto the rim of a conventional ashtray. A cigarette is held firmly in the ring so that ash falls safely into the ashtray. The filter tip of the cigarette is connected to the end of a gastric probe approximately twenty centimeters in length, which is connected in turn to a rectal probe of about the same length. The plastic tip at the end of this tube becomes the new filter for the smoker who can inhale their smoke thanks to this pseudo-hookah made of various found objects from the institute's supply cupboards. The ashtray thereby constructed, stamped with the name of its owner, is screwed into a table. Thus, even at an advanced stage and despite violent jerky motions, sick smokers can sit at tables on their balcony and enjoy a cigarette without running the risk of burning themselves or accidentally starting a fire.

It should now be clear, I hope, that at the Atlant Center care is not just about providing alternative treatment to Huntington's disease that would, itself, remain the same as it ever was. On the contrary, at Apeldoorn, another version of HD is cultivated and made real. What takes place is an intervention into its natural history, not only metaphorically but also in the strictly medical terms of its clinical course. This effect can be most clearly observed in relation to two symptoms, anosognosia and dementia. In the clinical literature, these come across as two more symptoms of a person with HD's lot. Anosognosia refers to a lack of self-awareness regarding symptoms and it is thought to be present, to a greater or lesser degree, throughout the entire evolution of the disease. As for dementia, it allegedly accompanies the condition's most advanced stages. What emerges, however, from discussions with caregivers at Apeldoorn is that none of them has observed either of these symptoms among residents. It is true, they say, that they grow slower and slower and that caregivers must have a great deal of patience to get answers to the questions they pose. But as to whether residents are anosognosic or demented, they answer no, not in the least. It is hard to resist the impression that if these symptoms are lacking it is above all because they are given no quarter at Apeldoorn, because HD patients are never addressed as if they were demented or anosognosic. Quite the opposite, staff at the Atlant Center always strive to take things from above, which is to say, to give as many opportunities as possible to their clients "to preserve, as much as can be, [their] capacity to act,"[25] to articulate themselves as actors in relation to what is happening to them – giving us a powerful and moving site of pragmatist morals and politics in action.[26]

25 Debaise, "La pensée laboratoire."
26 It must be noted that there is at least one important precursor to the care-philosophy practiced at Apeldoorn: The tireless US-American expert in HD-care, Jimmy Pollard – who has rendered his experiences public in a book called *Hurry-Up and Wait! A Cognitive Care Companion: Huntington's Disease in the Middle and more Advanced Years* (n.p.: Lulu.com, 2008).

Autonomy?

> *To the children [her nephews, who are all HD carri-*
> *ers], I say: be proud. You are extraordinary. You have*
> *a rare, unknown disease. You are extraordinary.*
> — Catherine[27]

From a historical standpoint, the autonomy concept, which is foundational to the right to know as well as to the concept of informed consent, is a consequence of mounting and warranted distrust of modern medicine and its practitioners. As described in previous chapters, since its very beginnings, the epistemological and methodological regime of modern medicine has tended to dissolve the bond between sick people and their conditions while, at the same time, placing distance between doctors and their patients. All too often, doctors treat sickness as a diagnostic entity (*disease*[28]) and not sick people themselves with their distinct and diverse experiences (*illness*[29]). This trajectory has been further cemented since the second half of the 20th century, with the technological know-how of intensive care, medical transplants, and reanimation. It reaches new heights with contemporary systems of social security and health insurance, which produce precise prescriptions of the quantum of financial support to be allocated to such and such a diagnosis, treatment option, or provision of care.

---

27 Excerpt from an interview conducted with Catherine, a woman from a family experiencing Huntington's across three generations. "Composer avec Huntington: La maladie de Huntington au soin de ses usagers," a report on exploratory research conducted between 2013–15 into experimental knowledge about HD, *Dingdingdong,* January 23, 2017, https://dingdingdong.org/a-propos/composer-avec-huntington/.

28 In English in the original text.

29 In English in the original text.

In the United States, as far back as the 1960s, a protest movement formed in response to an increasingly technological approach to medicine beholden to the laws of the market, dogmatic and "dehumanized," and giving less and less room to empathy, intimacy, or any acknowledgment of the values embedded within clinical acts. The new field of biomedical ethics was both the outcome and one of the driving forces behind this protest movement. It pushed for requirements concerning patient autonomy and the right to informed consent, which remain fundamental notions to this day. Autonomy emerged as the self-explanatory founding principle of a movement that followed in the footsteps of similar efforts within political and juridical circles. Guaranteeing patient autonomy, moreover, appeared to constitute a self-evident and robust response to mounting distrust of modern medicine: "Whereas trust had hitherto been the implicit moral understanding governing physician behavior and patient delegation of authority in the age of Johnson and Nixon, patient confidence required both new definition and novel substitutes."[30]

Nevertheless, upon closer inspection the autonomy concept is problematic in a number of different ways, sometimes even counterproductive. It rests upon an understanding of the patient that defers to the model of the rational, sovereign, and adult citizen, an individual who is able to decide and to act, consciously and with self-mastery – in other words, a non-relational being. Hence, to put it directly: the autonomy concept encourages tendencies within modern medicine identical to those it aims to critique. Indeed, "autonomy as configured in its individualistic stance facilitates the isolation required for positivism to operate freely."[31] Furthermore, bioethics

---

30 Alfred I. Tauber, *Patient Autonomy and the Ethics of Responsibility* (Cambridge: MIT Press, 2005), 43.
31 Ibid., 13.

discourse risks fashioning liberal subject-patients enti-tled to make rights claims against untrustworthy medi-cine, much like citizens would against the State. The dis-trust initially circulating among patients thus began to spread; doctors are now wary of their patients who have become possible future claimants. This is why doctors seek to protect themselves from the threat of legal action, which includes giving patients qua autonomous subjects a document detailing the risks accompanying treatment (for instance, a particular surgery) awaiting a signature as confirmation they have carefully read and understood it.

A similar reversal of fortunes occurred in relation to the patient's right to know, which is closely connected to the patient autonomy concept. In effect, this right tends to transform itself, surreptitiously, into an instruction or an imperative to know. Within this framework, a subject can only prove herself to be morally responsible if she transforms a genetic risk (e.g., the risk of having Hun-tington's or conditions such as high cholesterol, Alzhei-mer's, or various myopathies) into certainty. She does so by availing herself of testing and, accordingly, drawing conclusions as to appropriate life choices.

Another entity that emerged from dissatisfactions created by the health system has had, since the 1960s, a much more fascinating evolution in my view. This entity is the patients' association or, to be more accurate, pa-tients' collectives of a very particular sort: those whose actions go beyond fundraising for medical and pharma-ceutical research, which would otherwise limit them to operating within a resolutely hierarchical logic of knowl-edge production about a disease. Instead, they have opened the way to other forms of action that consist in cultivating their own skills in relation to the conditions that bring them together. We have already considered the example of the Hearing Voices Network. In recent dec-ades, Deaf people, Autistic people, the AIDS-movement, people with Parkinson's, and many others have increasingly organized collectively.[32] Heeding the call for "Nothing About Us Without Us," these movements place the user at the heart of their thinking and their actions – not in the sense of being a "consumer" of medical services but rather a co-constructor of the collective project of making a "user culture" for their given disease or difference of ability.

> The user culture, in contrast to instrumental, diagnostically justified uses, is a problem of collective interest that needs collective knowledge. We can call it a collective experience, in the old sense where the expertise first designates knowledge coming from experience and is cultivated in its relations with experience. [...] And this experience has a vital need for its own kind of knowledge that user associations can construct. This knowledge is valuable in itself, but in addition it can make other knowledges recognize that they are all gathered around something – a being? a power? – that belongs to no one, that no one can appropriate or represent.[33]

The making of such collective know-how about what is the liveliest life possible with a given condition does not necessarily aim at calling medical knowledge into question. Rather, it exists in addition to it, so as to rank among expert knowledge formations as a distinctive yet no less pertinent genre. Instead of placing themselves in the position of the victim, those engaged in such a task take

---

32 For questions concerning the movement and notion of disability pride, see Elisabeth Barnes, *The Minority Body* (Oxford: Oxford University Press, 2016). For more recent developments in disability studies, see Katie Ellis et al., eds., *Manifestos for the Future of Critical Disability Studies, Vol. 1* (London: Routledge, 2018) as well as the next volume by the same editors, *Interdisciplinary Approaches to Disability: Looking towards the Future* (London: Routledge 2018).

33 Stengers and Nathan, *Doctors and Healers*, 154–55.

charge, collectively, of setting the stage for their own future. And given the interest they grant themselves along with their own sickness or disability, given the manner in which they conjure ways of doing things with it, they also manage to awaken the interest of others as to what, from their perspective, matters most. This is what happens when psychiatrists ask for training from the Hearing Voices Network. The truth that such collectives bring to light is therefore not limited to their ability to draw attention to the tragedy of the disease or syndrome that befalls them. Rather, this truth appears "in the processes by which [these people] become, on their own terms, something other than victims; it is in their way of meddling with the processes that make victims out of them and thereby creating futures and fabulations rather than complaints or resentment."[34]

A brief outline of the Atlant Center allowed us to understand that both the autonomy concept and that of informed consent can hinder rather than help with situations of care. For care is precisely not developed in relation to an isolated subject but instead through a constant back-and-forth between patients, caregivers, doctors, and their kin, something that takes into account all of the actors and their various interests, needs, and interdependencies. None of them is, strictly speaking, autonomous. They each learn with and through one another, from within a strongly relational and co-constructed practice of care. Furthermore, the autonomy concept appears to be ill suited to what patient collectives such as voice hearers or people with Autism enact when, pointedly, they draw strength and energy from making what brings them together into a collective thing. At the risk of generalizing, it could be said that the autonomy concept tends to aim

---

34 "Une politique de l'hérésie. Entretien avec Isabelle Stengers," *Vacarme* 19, no. 2 (2002): 4–13, https://vacarme.org/article263.html. Translation mine.

either too high or too low. Too high, insofar as creating the necessary conditions for the relative wellbeing of sick people in care means repeatedly constraining their "autonomous" will, in the strong sense of the term. Too low, because the notion of informed consent, often used as a synonym for autonomy, falls short of the work of patient collectives who lay claim to a culture of their own making. If we are to retain the autonomy concept in spite of everything we have just considered, does it not follow that it should go hand in hand with the making of tools with which to think, tools that might help put medical knowledge in its place (*relativiser*), in the literal sense of connecting this know-how to other know-how making practices like those of user groups?

What Do the Oracles Tell Us?

> *A divinatory apparatus is always a creative act.*
> *It institutes the interface among universes; it*
> *makes them palpable and then thinkable.*
> – Tobie Nathan[35]

Comparisons with ancient oracles and seers often arise unprompted in discussions about testing for HD and other techniques of predictive testing. Media representations frequently draw on such imagery when describing and analyzing genetic knowledge about the future. It comes up regularly, however, in specialist literature as well. Consider, for example, that in 2001, before the completion of the human genome project, the German parliamentary committee evaluating the consequences of this technology produced a report titled *The Genetic Oracle: An Overview of Current Usage of Genetic Testing for Prognosis and Diagnosis*. Leading HD researchers themselves make use of images of oracles and divination to think through

35 Stengers and Nathan, *Doctors and Healers*, 10

the kind of knowledge they deal with and bring forth. Hence, between 1983 and 1993, Nancy Wexler published at least three articles on predictive genetic testing for HD whose very titles drew this connection: "The Oracle of DNA," "Clairvoyance and Caution," and "The Tiresias Complex."[36] Here is how the last of these, published in 1992, begins: "The blind seer Tiresias confronted Oedipus with the quintessential dilemma of modern genetics: 'It is but sorrow to be wise when wisdom profits not.'"[37]

All of these references index the tragedy predicted by ancient prophetic practices, the curses they would produce and human powerlessness before them. The association, therefore, is an almost exclusively negative or pejorative one. In this book's final section, I wish to pursue a hunch that oracular practices and predictive medicine might be connected in deeper, more interesting ways than these metaphorical transpositions suggest. I submit that a closer look at ancient oracles can heighten our sensitivity and provide instruction as we face up to the challenge of constructing a milieu better suited to welcoming the creature of predictive testing. Making this claim intelligible means following in the footsteps of the concrete practices of oracles. Specifically, we must pay the utmost attention to the many precautions and trials attached to oracular predictions, and which surrounded all those at Delphi and other sites where knowledge of the future was produced and relayed.

36 Nancy Wexler, "The Oracle of DNA," in *Molecular Genetics in Diseases of Brain, Nerve, and Muscle,* eds. L.P. Rowland et al. (Oxford: Oxford University Press, 1989), 429–42; Nancy Wexler, "Clairvoyance and Caution: Repercussions from the Human Genome Project," in *The Code of Codes: Scientific and Social Issues in the Human Genome Project,* eds. Daniel J. Kevles and Leroy Hood (Cambridge: Harvard University Press, 1992), 211–43; Nancy Wexler, "The Tiresias Complex: Huntington's Disease as a Paradigm of Testing for Late-Onset Disorders," *FASEB Journal* 6, no. 10 (1992): 2820–25.

37 Wexler, "The Tiresias Complex," 2820.

The most effective way of bringing into view the pivotal role that precautions played in the construction of
prophetic knowledge within ancient divination practices
is, without doubt, to recount what happens when consulting an oracle fails. Sometime in the 80s or early 90s of
the first century, a tragic accident took place in the temple of Apollo at Delphi, leading to the death of the Pythia, the high priestess who transmitted the word of the
deity. During a consultation with the oracle, the Pythia
began screaming and yelling as if possessed, and rushed
out of the temple's innermost shrine, the *adyton,* toward
the exit. She died a few days afterward. This incident
provoked considerable emotion among the residents of
Delphi. It deeply disturbed the temple's servants as well
as families in the city who entrusted their daughters to
the temple to be become Pythias. This, at least, is the
conclusion Plutarch comes to in *On the Obsolescence of the
Oracles,* his friend Nicander having held the priesthood
in the sanctuary at the time. Clearly very affected despite
the many intervening years, he recalls the incident as follows:

> Finally she became hysterical and with a frightful
> shriek rushed towards the exit and threw herself down,
> with the result that not only the members of the dep-
> utation fled, but also the oracle-interpreter Nicander
> and those holy men that were present. However, after
> a little, they went in and took her up, still conscious;
> and she lived on for a few days.[38]

---

38 Plutarch, *Moralia, Volume V: Isis and Osiris. The E at Delphi. The Oracles
at Delphi No Longer Given in Verse. The Obsolescence of Oracles,* trans.
Frank Cole Babbitt (Cambridge: Harvard University Press, 1936), 499.
My analysis builds on historian Dominique Jaillard's examination of
this incident in Plutarch's moral writings. See Dominique Jaillard,
"Plutarque et la divination: La piété d'un prêtre philosophe," *Revue
de l'histoire des religions* 2 (2007): 149–69.

What culminates in this dramatic event? What events led up to it? What caused the Pythia's violent and terrifying unraveling, which horrified those present and chased them from the temple, and brought about the Pythia's own demise? Plutarch, who himself would later enter the Delphic priesthood and practice for some thirty years, goes beyond mere conjecture. In his judgment, the Pythia's death is the clear and direct effect of an infringement committed by the temple's servants against the rules of the sacrificial ritual preceding consultation.

> As it happened, a deputation from abroad had arrived to consult the oracle. The victim, it is said, remained unmoved and unaffected in any way by the first libations; but the priests, in their eagerness to please, went far beyond their wonted usage, and only after the victim had been subjected to a deluge and nearly drowned did it at last give in.[39]

As often happened at Delphi, a delegation went to the temple to ask the oracle about matters of State. What's more, it would appear that the envoys enjoyed the privilege of consulting the Pythia before everyone else who had come seeking advice. There was an evident desire to not disappoint these important political figures by making them wait for a subsequent consultation, even though the signs were not favorable, meaning that the divinatory powers of the Pythia were compromised.

The so-called preliminary rituals, the preparations and preliminary precautions taken before all consultations with the Pythia, had an essential place and significance within Delphic liturgy. They entailed a series of steps that bring into full relief the deep sacredness of any act of divination, an act demanding cautious and attentive preparation and accompaniment. The first of these

39 Plutarch, *Moralia, Volume V,* 499.

Delphic preliminaries was setting the date of consultation. Whereas, in the oracle's early years, "it was but once a year, on the god Apollo's birthday, when the oracles were given,"[40] a more frequent tempo was later observed. Thereafter, the Pythia could be consulted on the seventh day of each month and, in summer, on the days following as well. "In addition to this, it was also possible to arrange 'special meetings,' always on condition that the sacrifices were favorable and thus indicated that the god was ready to form a relationship with the priestess."[41] To ensure that the signs were favorable and that the oracle could be "operational," so to speak, before all consultations an animal would be offered in sacrifice. However, other rituals preceded this step, rituals during which each animal was subjected to a specific trial that served to determine whether or not it was to be sacrificed.

> For what is to be offered in sacrifice must, both in body and in soul, be pure, unblemished, and unmarred. Indications regarding the body it is not at all difficult to perceive, but they test the soul by setting meal before the bulls and peas before the boars; and the animal that does not eat of this they think is not of sound mind. In the case of the goat, they say, cold water gives positive proof; for indifference and immobility against being suddenly wet is not characteristic of a soul in a normal state.[42]

If the goat flinched, its neck hair standing on end, if the bull ate the meal or the boar the peas, only then was it possible to conclude that the signs were favorable for a consultation. The sacrifice could only commence once

---

40 Marion Giebel, *Das Orakel von Delphi. Geschichte und Texte* (Stuttgart: Reclam, 2001), 16. Translation mine.

41 Ibid.

42 Plutarch, *The Obsolescence of Oracles*, 495.

the animal had given its consent by way of these signs. The Pythia was then in a position to make contact with the god Apollo and he, for his part, was ready to confer the requisite predisposition upon the priestess, namely the "inspiration" or breath he transferred to her. Nevertheless, before she could truly be interrogated, those who came seeking advice had also to submit to a series of preliminary rituals. They had to purify themselves, burn a sacred wafer, and, at a later period, give an offering to the priest for another prior sacrifice. Only upon completing all of these rituals were they admitted into the adyton of the temple of Apollo. Finally, the Pythia herself had to undertake a series of ritual acts before assuming her position atop the tripod in the temple. "She would take a ritual bath in the Castalian Spring, drink the waters of the Cassotis, chew laurel leaves and light incense"[43] These preparatory measures were integral to undertaking the Delphic oracle. The sacrifices themselves had a divinatory value, indexing whether the conditions were right for allowing the Pythia to fulfill her function and, with Apollo's aid, answer the questions brought before her. If one of the conditions was not met, no demand should rightfully take place.

> Whenever, then, the imaginative and prophetic faculty is in a state of proper adjustment for attempering itself to the spirit as to a drug, inspiration in those who foretell the future is bound to come; and whenever the conditions are not thus, it is bound not to come, or when it does come to be misleading, abnormal, and confusing.[44]

On the day when the Pythia fled the *adyton* in the middle of a consultation, the goats awaiting sacrifice failed,

43 Giebel, *Das Orakel von Delphi*, 18
44 Plutarch, *The Obsolescence of Oracles*, 499.

as Plutarch told us, to flinch. Despite this, the temple's servants took the risk of authorizing the consultation. No sooner had the session begun than those present took note of the Pythia's disturbed inspiration:

> She went down into the oracle unwillingly, they say, and half-heartedly; and at her first responses it was at once plain from the harshness of her voice that she was not responding properly; she was like a labouring ship and was filled with a mighty and baleful spirit.[45]

This story exposes the dangers of trying to conjure fore-knowledge by forcing a laboring Pythia to take up her position within the holy of holies. The gift of "the imaginative faculty" or of divine inspiration then swiftly becomes a poison. This pharmacological quality of the foretelling of future events draws successful colloquy with the divine and its failed and death-dealing counterpart into striking proximity, the two separated by a mere difference in dosage. Promising prediction (*maintain*) and speech that is uninspired, mad, and dangerous (*mania*) are frightfully close to one another. Divinatory art's Janus face was constitutive of the Delphic oracle's protocol.

> It is for these reasons that they guard the chastity of the priestess, and keep her life free from all association and contact with strangers, and take the omens before the oracle, thinking that it is clear to the god when she has the temperament and disposition suitable to submit to the inspiration without harm to herself.[46]

In such light, any consultation with the Pythia came with the additional risk of unraveling the relationship between a god (or goddess) and his (or her) prophet (or

45 Ibid.
46 Ibid., 501.

prophetess), this latter being the one who speaks (-*phete*) for (*pro*-) another, who speaks in their name. For even on days when the signs were favorable and when the Pythia did not resemble "a labouring ship [...] filled with a mighty and baleful spirit," it was clear to see that the labor of divination was, as Plutarch explains, exhausting: "the Pythia regains calm and tranquility once she has left her tripod and its exhalations."[47] The duty of the priest and the rest of the temple's servants was to make sure that the risky relationship between the god Apollo and the Pythia, between divine foresight and its foretelling, would unfold as serenely as could be. This presumed following the liturgical rules to the letter. Forcing the Pythia to answer a question, to foretell the future and offer advice, despite all of the signs indicating she was incapable of responding (that she was, literally, *ir-respons-able*) was, therefore, playing with death.

It is easy to imagine that the broken rules that lead to the Pythia's death not only endangered the seer's existence but everyone else's as well. On one hand, because the consultants would endeavor, after the consultation had concluded, to ensure that their actions, whether personal or political, lined up with the oracle's "harshly" spoken words. This alone could produce fatal consequences in some cases. It was not unheard of, for instance, for the Delphic oracle to influence major decisions about warfare. On the other, wild and demonic divine entities had thus been unleashed, without having been tempered or tamed by ritual techniques; they had been provoked by transgressions of those rules that should have been respected when making contact with divine beings. The danger was therefore that they, in turn, would violently

47 Plutarch. *Moralia, Volume IX: Table-Talk, Books 7–9. Dialogue on Love,* trans. Edwin L. Minar, F.H. Sandbach, and W.C. Helmbold (Cambridge: Harvard University Press, 1961), 365–67.

take possession of those who had invoked them. The danger, in other words, was becoming possessed.

Other oracular practices were subject to strict rules and called for circumspect usage. Whether it was observing birds in flight, interpreting the motion of oil beads on the water's surface, or reading the entrails of animals sacrificed for fortunetelling, "advising was a skill that corresponded to a reading ability."[48] This ability needed to be learned carefully. Entrails, for instance, were cast in clay or bronze and stamped with the correct marking. Novices could practice anatomy on these and also pursue inquiries into the correspondences between micro-signs read in the entrails and their implications for the world.

> As in medical discourse, the symptoms were condensed into diagnoses and the diagnoses into prognoses. [...] The results were to be analyzed and carefully preserved. Indeed, it was not unusual that an advisor who erred would earn cruel punishment. According to a story related by Herodotus, among the Scythians, failed seers were strapped to a cattle cart and burned alive using bundles of willow branches, the same material with which they would practice divination.[49]

In light of the threat brought about through false prediction, "advisors tried, very early on, to dissociate the quality of their advice from the consequences of the actions they recommended."[50] For this reason, most of the time at Delphi and elsewhere, advice and prophecy took the form of a riddle. Doing so ensured that the prediction would be followed by an interpretive phase, one for which the

---

48 Thomas Macho, "Was tun? Skizzen zur Wissensgeschichte der Beratung," in *Think Tanks: Die Beratung der Gesellschaft*, eds. Thomas Brandstetter, Claus Pias, and Sebastian Vehlken (Berlin: Diaphanes, 2010), 59–85, at 63. Translation mine.

49 Ibid., 64.

50 Ibid., 65.

oracle itself had no responsibility. The advice was disso-
ciated in two steps: "first came the giving of transcend-
ent, charismatic, or medium-like commentary and then
came the interpretation of this commentary."[51] While the
actual seer (e.g., the Pythia or the Sybil whom the gods
inspired) spoke in riddles, a whole host of specialists in
reading, translating, and interpreting riddling speech
acts stood at the ready around Delphi and in other oracular places. A real prophecy only acquired its meaning and
momentum once it had passed through many hands: after it became, as it were, collectivized. In so doing, it was
imperative that the proper division of labor was maintained, for this simultaneously distributed responsibility
for the ensuing prediction. In this context, the production of ever-fragile foreknowledge therefore relied upon
the strategic proliferation of actors and functions, for
both preliminary and subsequent purposes. Without the
coordinated intervention of these various roles, it would
not, in fact, be possible to produce this knowledge at all.

The oracles therefore draw our attention to at least
two aspects of diagnostic predictions. First, whenever
a predictive practice allows itself to subject the person
questioning the oracle to scrupulous examination without taking into consideration the concrete circumstances of the ecological situation, it will inevitably become
extremely dangerous. In addition, while it is true that
informed production of knowledge about the future requires prophetic speech, at the same time, it calls for a
sophisticated and technically refined interpretive art.
Plutarch's description of the Pythia's death offers a striking demonstration. This analysis takes on a particular
contemporary hue if we consider it in relation to non-
Western divinatory healing practices, whether ancient or
contemporary. For these practices do not pin symptoms
onto the sick person but instead always attribute them

51 Ibid.

to beings requiring careful identification.[52] A "diagnosis" corresponds, above all, to the identification of such a being: what is its nature, what are its intentions, how might it be tamed? The answers to these questions are integral to the treatment and rely as much on the healer's expertise as the cultural group to whom the latter belongs. As such, there is no difference in kind between diagnosis, prognosis, and treatment in such a framework. They form an ensemble involved in ever-renewed ways of collectively practicing the demanding art of negotiating with the invisible.[53]

Plutarch's text engages a broader set of concerns. A series of interlocutors who happen to be at Delphi give voice to Plutarch's own thoughts on the matter. These various interlocutors assemble to examine the reasons why, unlike what happened under the Greeks, oracles began disappearing one-by-one during Roman rule. Decreasing population in the areas of major oracular sites would have led to a more limited demand for their services, but also to the withdrawal of the beings in charge (*daimones*) from their sanctuaries. We would have "unlearned" how to correctly handle the oracle along the way, much like we forget how to use a musical instrument that we leave idle too long. The Pythia – whose speech reveals a "harshness of her voice" and who rushed out of the temple like a fury – only comes up towards the close of this wider discussion. In the most striking manner, she embodies the dangers that threaten to arise from a lack of collective attention to a phenomenon as volatile as foreknowledge. Oracular practice of the kind Plutarch describes is,

---

52 To be sure, this manner of separating a person from her symptoms is in no way to be confused with the separation of patients and their diseases as described by Canguilhem. Rather, the separation in question relies on an entirely different model of patients, pathologies, and their relation to one another.

53 Nathan and Stengers, *Doctors and Healers*. See also Tobie Nathan, *L'étranger ou le pari de l'autre* (Paris: Éditions Autrement, 2014).

in our view, a precedent when it comes to the ecology of diagnostic prediction. The Pythia's death, in this sense, is an ecological crisis.

Conclusion

This book began with a twofold challenge. The first was to go beyond the critical perspective that Alice Rivières vehemently established as she apprehended the violence inherent in diagnosis as more than the failure of a particular doctor or institution. Our task, instead, was to make sense of it as the effect of a given epistemological and deontological regime. The second challenge was to resist the widespread notion that new techniques come into being with already stabilized, clearly defined problems, and that our mandate was to react by taking ethical and legal measures like setting protocols, establishing terms of accessibility, and other guidelines.

To depart from this approach, I suggested we take up an ecological perspective that would force us to elaborate well-constructed problems in relation to the new technical entities that inhabit our world. These problems would allow us to establish more constructive relationships with these entities. On this basis, rather than knowing whether a technique is in itself admissible or not, the question becomes one of knowing how we might assemble ecological milieus or situations fostering the existence of the conditions needed to most assuredly and effectively welcome an entity like the creature commonly known as the "predictive test."

Yet modern medicine – in the name of the scientific recognition to which it aspired – separated the sick person from the disease and thus interrupted the doctor–patient relationship. At the same time, it drew upon a radical epistemological separation of facts from values in order to delegitimize any modes of access to disease deemed "unscientific" by modern standards. There is little room for the patients' perspective within this kind of medicine. What such perspectives might contribute to diagnosis as well as to therapeutic decisions must, in keeping with this logic, remain at a minimum. Only in this way could medicine achieve and sustain its aspiration to scientific rationality, which is to say, to the systematic universalization of medical knowledge. Within a system like this, the patient or anyone else lacking medical qualifications, no matter how profound their connection to the illness, is denied from working towards fashioning a given disease on the basis of experience or artistic, historical, or philosophical know-how. For as we have seen, to put it in the plainest terms, the very people touched by disease are, strictly speaking, no longer the objects of medicine. This is especially due to the increasingly dominant role ascribed to quantitative methods within health. Coinciding with the emergence of the 19th-century social hygiene movement, the close connection between medicine and statistical knowledge gradually imposed itself upon all its domains. So-called "evidence-based medicine" has continued this tradition, and since the 1990s, statistically derived (and therefore unimpeachable) knowledge has been elevated to the rank of the central truth criterion.

Taken to its limit, it can be said that from a statistical point of view the patient is not a person. They are not somebody but rather, following Tobie Nathan, *anybody*

(*quiconque*).¹ The regime of modern medicine is intimate-
ly entwined with this practice of *anybodification*. When
the doctor foretells that the "verdict" Alice receives of "44
CAG repetitions" will be "unbearable," this speech act can
be understood as the effect of the statistical transformation of a person into an anybody. It is a form of proof-
making that surreptitiously shifts from constative utterance ("44") to performative utterance ("unbearable"). The
two kinds of utterance merge through this operation,
dissembling a fundamental point: the term "unbearable"
refers to a statistical monstrosity whereby *anybody* presenting forty-four repetitions will have an unbearable future. And yet such a statement fails to account for Alice's
actual and concrete future.

Stephen J. Gould offers perhaps the most compelling
account of the traps and devastating effects to which
statistics give rise in relation to life-changing diagnoses.
In a short piece eloquently titled "The Median Isn't the
Message," Gould writes that in 1982 he learned he "was
suffering from abdominal mesothelioma, a rare and serious cancer."² He then decided to review the latest literature on this form of cancer. "The literature couldn't
have been more brutally clear: mesothelioma is incurable, with a median mortality of only eight months after discovery."³ Then, Gould explains, he used his understanding of the purposes and limits of statistics, learned
from evolutionary biology, to convince himself that this
scientifically founded information did not mean, as one
generally presumes, that he would invariably cease liv-

---

1   Tobie Nathan, "En psychothérapie: maladies, patients, sujets, clients
    ou usagers?" paper presented at *La psychothérapie à l'épreuve de ses
    usagers*, Centre Devereux, Paris, France, October 12, 2006. Available
    online at http://www.ethnopsychiatrie.net/tobieusagers.htm
2   Stephen Jay Gould, "The Median Isn't the Message," in *The Richness of
    Life: The Essential Stephen Jay Gould*, eds. Paul McGarr and Steven Rose
    (New York: Norton, 2006), 26–31, at 27.
3   Ibid.

ing in eight months' time. His main argument is that our Platonic heritage, with its emphasis on clear distinctions and firm boundaries, beguiles us into radically misinterpreting statistical studies – "opposite to the appropriate interpretation in our actual world of variation, shadings, and continua."[4] Instead of considering variations as the "hard realities" and means and medians as abstractions, our customary view of things has us take up the polar opposite position. We are used to conceiving of "means and medians as the hard 'realities,' and the variation that permits their calculation as a set of transient and imperfect measurements of this hidden essence."[5] Therein lies our fundamental mistake, a mistake that comes with an existential threat. In effect, when "the median is the reality and variation around the median just a device for its calculation, the 'I will probably be dead in eight months' may pass as a reasonable interpretation."[6] Statistics, it is plain to see, are a total abstraction translated into numbers. It is therefore from the perspective of science itself that the narrative hold they have over the individual must be called into question. We must do away with the habit of automatically turning means and medians into proof, deemed valid for a given concrete case such that its distinctiveness is not taken into account, not even gesturally or provisionally. In effect, if we emphasize variations, the only person whose life expectancy is reduced to eight months is an anybody, an anybody who only exists in the statistical realm.

In this sense, the task of elaborating a milieu that is capable of welcoming our creature, the "predictive test" for HD, is above all one of resisting the hold of the anybody. From within this context, resisting this hold assumes the ability to become able to recognize that test

4   Ibid., 28.
5   Ibid.
6   Ibid.

results which appear to take an abstract form, such as the number "44," are not explanatory but instead, because they address a concrete person, are first and foremost a riddle. What is to be done, then, is to take care of this riddle together and, along the way, take lesson from the proliferating becomings contained within.

Afterword

Isabelle Stengers

I am writing this afterword as almost ten years have passed since the founding of Dingdingdong, the Institute for the Coproduction of Knowledge about Huntington's Disease. Initiated by Emilie Hermant and Valérie Pihet, both Katrin Solhdju and myself are among its members. This collective began its adventure following Alice Rivières's early encounters with a medical establishment that proved to be in complete disarray in the face of Huntington's disease, its definitions, its incurability, its heredity, and its predictive testing. In 2013, Alice Rivières recounted this experience in *The Dingdingdong Manifesto*, the inaugural publication of the Éditions Dingdingdong publishing house. Two years later, Éditions Dingdingdong published the French edition of *Testing Knowledge*. These two texts make up the present volume.

Founding the Dingdingdong Collective turned out to be a transformative experience for all of its members, whatever their practice. This is because Dingdingdong creates an understanding of these same practices such that they warrant the interest of the virtual community concerned with, attached to, or connected through the questions Huntington's disease raises. Joining Dingdingdong therefore involves actively and creatively situating ourselves as a part of this community, as subjects touched by these questions.

Katrin Solhdju's *Testing Knowledge* is the work of a historian and epistemologist of medicine and its experimental practices. However – and this is no contradiction – it is also a book committed to, thought through, and written "in the presence" of people who have decided to take the genetic test that stands to identify them as carriers or non-carriers of the genetic mutation responsible for Hungtington's disease. It puts into question a diagnosis, one whose predictive power is matched only by the disarray it causes; because, in this instance, for every call of "now that we can know," there is never a corresponding "here's what we can do." In medicine, the idea that once a "cause" is identified then treatment follows is alive and well. Research is ongoing. Its temporal horizon, however, is too far off to enable those who pronounce the diagnosis to follow it with words of hope and encouragement (or the prospect of good news to come).

When reduced to a "fact" – you're either a carrier or you aren't – diagnosis can crush the very person who wanted to know. As she explains in *The Dingdingdong Manifesto,* Alice Rivières experienced the announcement of her test results as an extremely violent verdict. The doctor knows what will happen to her, and this knowledge brooks no appeal. She cannot do anything but await the inevitable, the onset of the first symptoms that mark the beginning of a slow decline. Solhdju reminds us that we use the word "prophet" to refer to someone who speaks in the name of a power that legitimates or authorizes their discourse. The doctor prophesizes in the name of the power of scientific truth, but it is a truth that deprives Alice of any possible hold on her own life, because medicine has no hold over the disease. Dindingdong was created, as a collective, on the basis of Alice's refusal to let this knowledge crush her. It is not a matter of denying its truth, but rather, of repopulating the world that it depleted.

Solhdju argues for an ecology of diagnosis, that is to say, for an approach that does not separate diagnosis from the milieu that confers meaning upon it and lends it consequence. It is worth emphasizing that such an approach is not *critical* in the sense of aiming to reduce diagnosis to a mere function of its milieu. Coming from someone who treats people, a diagnosis is *agentive,* it is a vector of transformation in and of itself, and as such has a stake in the art of healing. Hence, the milieu does not explain diagnosis. Rather, it achieves its explanation *through* diagnosis. For Solhdju, the ecological approach "problematizes" because it excludes any position of exteriority or detachment. It seeks to "posit" a problem "well." This does not mean making the problem go away, but rather, deploying it in a mode through which it acquires irreducible bearing and significance.

You might say that Solhdju offers her own response to the call Bruno Latour made in his landmark article "Why Has Critique Run Out of Steam?" After glossing the ways in which the "merchants of doubt" captured and repurposed the critical approach, he asks: "Can we devise another powerful descriptive tool that deals this time with matters of concern and whose import then will no longer be to debunk but to protect and care, as Donna Haraway would put it? Is it really possible to transform the critical urge in the ethos of someone who *adds* reality to matters of fact and not *subtracts* reality?"[1]

This is no coincidence but the trace of a common commitment: whether it is the "fact" that climate scientists' observations and models allow for a conclusion about manmade climate disruption or the "fact" that particular genetic traits allow for the predictive diagnosis of Huntington's, each requires commitment as a "matter of concern" but this does not mean simply yielding or deferring to them. They must take on a greater reality than the ab-

---

1   Bruno Latour, "Why Has Critique Run out of Steam? From Matters of Fact to Matters of Concern," *Critical Inquiry* 30, no. 2 (2004): 225–48, at 232.

stract reality of "Q.E.D." For facts like these say nothing about the consequences of their demonstration. Indeed, it is in this sense that they differ from the "experimental fact." Solhdju reminds us that the experimental fact's success hinges on the possibility of the experimenter withdrawing, avowing that the experimental set-up allows the phenomenon under investigation to "speak for itself." However, the people it addresses, other experimenters, do not *suffer* a verdict. Rather, they are *concerned*: they go on to explore the consequences of their colleagues' success, which is to say they *augment* its reality.

Solhdju's ecological approach draws a strong distinction between the respective milieus of the "experimental fact" and the "clinical fact," even though so-called "evidence-based" medicine insists on their common ancestry. Facts are "agentive" in both instances; they prompt action, although not in the same way. However, this claim to common ancestry is itself agentive. This is because the doctor does not take on the role of mediator, of someone who creates a putatively therapeutic relationship between the patient and "the facts" by "adding" something to "the facts" such that they become the centerpiece of a healing process. Instead, the doctor plays the role of mere intermediary, that is to say, of the spokesperson for a verdict wrought from another order of knowledge altogether, so-called objective knowledge, which characterizes what "objectively" ails the patient.[2] Of course, the doctor can profess their confidence in a given course of treatment, the effectiveness of which is also grounded in "facts," and it is assumed that they always behave "humanely." However, they can go no further. Another agen-

---

2   A central distinction Bruno Latour has introduced is the difference between an intermediary, an entity that loyally translates relations but does not transform them, and a mediator, an entity that has the capacity to create relations and transform them. See Bruno Latour, *Reassembling the Social: An Introduction to Actor-Network Theory* (Oxford: Oxford University Press, 2005), 39.

tive figure haunts the stage: the charlatan. Their art runs the risk of producing therapeutic effects reminiscent of medicine's shameful past.

Within this milieu – which requires that the doctor, lest they pass for a charlatan, be a loyal intermediary and refrain from adding anything to the facts that might commit them to a healing relationship – the predictive diagnosis for Huntington's disease is a disturbance that gives rise to what Solhdju terms an "ecological crisis." It is as if the novel entity's very presence is disordering and, barring a disastrous turn of events, calls for the problematization of roles and positions. In following Nancy Wexler and referring to this entity as "the creature," she irresistibly turns our thoughts toward Frankenstein's creature, that unfortunate being hated by its creator and whom this hatred, the father's refusal to invent a way of welcoming it, turned evil.

How can the Hippocratic oath's call to "do no harm," the doctor's primary duty, combine with the effective malevolence that this loyal intermediary must present as factual information? The doctor may claim that doing no harm in this instance means respecting the autonomous subject who must confront the naked truth, i.e., find the inner resources needed to mourn any hope of leading a normal life. However, with a curious sleight of hand, the intermediary then transforms themself into conscience's guide. They direct the patient to give up on the fantasy of consolation "for their own good." This is, to be sure, an ecological crisis: a fact becomes a duty.

The Dingdingdong collective does not take blame as its vocation. However, it wagers that narratives other than decline without remedy and experiences other than irretrievable displacement and fractured relationships exist and can, when activated, become agentive, repopulating the imaginations of people concerned with Huntington's disease. They may be carriers, sick persons, loved ones, or medical and paramedical caregivers; we name them "users," because the task is to cultivate "usages," ways of doing and building relations. This is Solhdju's wager. Nothing will make the telling of a "positive" genetic test result something other than an ordeal (*épreuve*) – a testing experience for the person who thereafter knows they are a carrier, for their loved ones, and also for the doctor who has to make the announcement. The "creature," however, remains silent about the nature of this ordeal. What speaks in their name is, above all, the doctor's knowledge of medicine's powerlessness.

In a video produced by Dingdingdong in 2013, this doctor's name is Marboeuf, and he recounts his confrontation with Alice Rivières's sister who reproaches him for not having said that he did not know. Yes, she allows, there may be statistics, but they are just as silent about what will happen to her sister *in particular*. Giving voice, as Solhdju observes, to those to whom the ordeal is presented as something to which they will be subjected, when it is in fact *the doctor* who is subjected to *medicine*'s powerlessness to act, Rivières' sister adds: "The truth of our disease does not belong to you or, at any rate, at least not *only* to you." This presents an opportunity to propose a speculative narrative. What if, instead of buttressing his clear conscience as "someone who is no charlatan, who sticks to the facts," Doctor Marboeuf took an interest in the way that elsewhere (e.g., in the Netherlands) the "truth of medicine" exists only in caregiving, in spatial arrangements, in inventing techniques for enabling life, modes of attention, as a range of ways of doing everything possible to "dedramatize" this sickness? Hence, another ecology of illness would be possible, an ecology that would multiply agentive systems, not to produce miracles but rather to give living well a chance.

These days, a whole range of user groups are taking shape, some with doctors and some without, creating new milieus, to forge new ecologies for the sicknesses that ail them or to "depathologize" the singular disorder with which they live. Hence, voice hearers refuse to accept that their voices belong to schizophrenia as a psychopathological category. As for Dingdingdong, we reject the term "neurodegenerative" as applied to Huntington's disease, we can accept the term "neuroevolutive," yet refuse to isolate the neurological from the relationships that come together or fall apart within its multiple milieus. Can we really imagine a doctor turning an unfavorable test result into the revelation of a metamorphic future and the need to "prepare the soul" so that this metamorphosis goes "as well as it can, despite the intense turbulence it will not fail to bring about"?[3]

Can we also imagine that a doctor, reading the final pages of Solhdju's book, would seriously consider the connection she ventures to draw with the oracular practices of the Pythia at Delphi? For the Pythia was also an intermediary, yet she belonged to a world in which people knew that contact between her and her god ran the risk of destructive possession and that ritual precautions were necessary for her own safety. It was also known that naked prophetic speech was dangerous, requiring that mediators intercede and interpret it. Today, the oracles are gone but seers do still exist. One such person, Maud Kristen, agreed to extend the speculative story of Doctor Marboeuf by addressing a letter to him. The following is an excerpt:

Your practices, like mine, question the future and interpret data using various markers.

You question and interpret samples, as do I... Your media are blood or secretions. Mine are initials, images, cards, or photographs. Divination or medical ex-

---

3 See "Composer avec Huntington: La maladie de Huntington au soin de ses usagers," *Dingdingdong*, January 23, 2017, https://dingding-dong.org/a-propos/composer-avec-huntington/.

aminations deliver verdicts. But haven't you forgotten that only your patient or my client turns this verdict into a "destiny"? Haven't you forgotten that they are in no way reducible to the bad news afflicting them?

You and I, Doctor, we both own a diagnosis. That's all. That's quite a lot already. But we never own what they will weave from their "bad news," never what their life will become after the announcement, nor the sense they will or won't make of all this.

No point, therefore, trying to convince them that everything is done for. The only thing that's done for is perhaps or probably, I concede, life as an able person for much longer, but it's not the man or woman you have before you and about whom you know nothing.[4]

For Katrin Solhdju, the historian and epistemologist, the question of predictive diagnosis for Huntington's disease forced her to vacate her analytical position, not to abandon its rigor but rather its presumed detachment. She had to give this question the form of a riddle that compels thinking and imagining. What this meant, she notes, was going "one step further to interrogate the propositional potential of [her own] conceptual, historical, and empirical research." In order to "posit the problem well," to give it a reality that might be shared with those concerned with this problem, she dared to take seriously the question that the presymptomatic test for Huntington's disease raises. This is not one of prediction in general but the question of people who "tell the future," who tell a person's future when asked. The fact that Solhdju queries what makes someone capable of this – whether that is

4   Maud Kristen, "Lettre de Maud Kristen au Dr Marboeuf," Dingding-dong, March 1, 2015, https://dingdingdong.org/departements/narration-speculative/lettre-de-maud-kristen-au-dr-marboeuf/.

genetics, cards, photographs, or the Pythia's god Apollo – is not a sign of disrespect or irreverence, it shows no desire to scandalize those for whom only medical prediction is objective. The question is not what authorizes such knowledge but the ordeal (*épreuve*) it enacts. What is specific about the situation of the doctor announcing test results is, perhaps, that the ecology of the medical milieu is unfavorable to the culture of protection that the "foreteller's" position requires and to the multiplication of mediators necessary to add reality to the genetic "fact."

In Alice Rivières's case, the medical team's preoccupation turned on the following question: can the person who asks to know withstand the telling of a future that will one day be theirs? This is a bad question, as the genetic fact is not "their" future. However, it is a question that articulates the intermediary's drama: what they have to foretell may lead to suicide, but the intermediary can only impart this knowledge in all its horror.

Of course, Solhdju's ecological approach does not call for doctors to become possessed by a divine force or to learn how to read cards. But it does call for the coproduction of all kinds of knowledge and practice that make up the landscape awaiting the carrier. It calls for doctors to not leave the recipient of "bad news" alone before the desert of a life deprived of possibility, to add to this news some gesture of interest in a landscape of possible relations, encounters, futures, and histories. Such is the landscape that will give truth to diagnosis, the truth of a life that can be lived well all the same.

Bibliography

Ageron, Pierre. "Le partage des dix-sept chameaux et autres arithmétiques attributes à l'immam 'Alî: Mouvance et circulation de récits de la tradition musulmane chiite." *Revue d'histoire des mathématiques* 19 (2013): 1–41. https://ageron.users.lmno.cnrs.fr/17chameaux.pdf.

Almqvist, Elisabeth W., Maurice Bloch, Ryan Brinkman, David Craufurd, and Michael R Hayden. "A Worldwide Assessment of the Frequency of Suicide, Suicide Attempts, or Psychiatric Hospitalization after Predictive Testing for Huntington's Disease." *The American Journal of Human Genetics* 64, no. 5 (May 1999): 1293–304. DOI: 10.1086/302374.

Austin, John L. *How to Do Things with Words.* Oxford: Oxford University Press, 1962.

Barnes, Elisabeth. *The Minority Body.* Oxford: Oxford University Press, 2016.

Bergson, Henri. *The Creative Mind: An Introduction to Metaphysics.* Translated by Mabelle Andison. Mineola: Dover Publications, 2007.

Bing, François, and Jean-François Braunstein. "Entretien avec Georges Canguilhem." *Interdisciplines* 1 (1984): 21–34.

Blanchot, Maurice. *The Book to Come.* Translated by Charlotte Mandell. Stanford: Stanford University Press, 2003.

Bucka-Lassen, Edlef. *Das schwere Gespräch. Patientengerechte Vermittlung einschneidender Diagnosen.* Cologne: Deutscher Ärzte-Verlag, 2005.

Canguilhem, Georges. *A Vital Rationalist: Selected Writings from Georges Canguilhem.* Edited by François Delaporte, translarted by Arthur Goldhammer. New York: Zone Books, 1993.

———. *Études d'histoire et de philosophie des sciences concernant les vivants et la vie.* Paris: Vrin, 2002.

———. *Writings on Medicine.* Translated by Stefanos Geroulanos and Todd Meyers. New York: Fordham University Press, 2012.

"Composer avec Huntington: La maladie de Huntington au soin de ses usagers." *Dingdingdong,* January 23, 2017. https://dingdingdong.org/a-propos/composer-avec-huntington/.

Debaise, Didier. "La pensée laboratoire: Une approche pragmatique de la connaissance." In *Éduquer dans le monde contemporain: Les savoirs et la société de la connaissance,* edited by Ali Benmakhlouf and Nicolas Piqué, 63–74. Casablanca: Le Fennec, 2013.

Debaise, Didier, Valérie Pihet, Katrin Solhdju, and Fabrizio Terranova "Speculative Narration: A Conversation with Valérie Pihet, Didier Debaise, Katrin Solhdju, and Fabrizio Terranova." *Parse* 7 (2017): 65–77. http://parsejournal.com/article/speculative-narration/.

Deleuze, Gilles. *Difference and Repetition.* Translated by Paul Patton. London and New York: Continuum, 1994.

Despret, Vinciane. *Our Emotional Makeup: Ethnopsychology and Selfhood.* New York: Other Press, 2004.

Ellis, Katie, Rosemarie Garland-Thomson, Mike Kent, and Rachel Robertson, eds. *Manifestos for the Future of Critical Disability Studies,* Vol. 1. London: Routledge, 2018.

———. *Interdisciplinary Approaches to Disability: Looking towards the Future.* London: Routledge, 2018.

"Ethical Issues Policy Statement on Huntington's Disease Molecular Genetics Predictive Test." *Journal of Medical Genetics* 27, no. 7 (1990): 34–38, DOI: 10.1136/jmg.27.1.34.

"Ethical Issues Policy Statement on Huntington's Disease Molecular Genetics Predictive Test." *Journal of the Neurological Sciences* 94, nos. 1–3 (1989): 327–32. DOI: 10.1016/0022-510X(89)90243-8.

Freemon, Frank R. "Pretesting for Huntington's Disease: Another View." *Hastings Center Report* 3, no. 4 (September 1973): 13. DOI: 10.2307/3561533.

Gaudillière, Jean-Paul. *La médecine et les sciences. XIXe et XXe siècles.* Paris: La Découverte, 2006.

Gehring, Petra. "Fragliche Expertise. Zur Etablierung von Bioethik in Deutschland." In *Wissenschaft und Demokratie,* edited by Michael Hagner, 112–39. Frankfurt am Main: Suhrkamp Verlag, 2012.

Giebel, Marion. *Das Orakel von Delphi. Geschichte und Texte.* Stuttgart: Reclam, 2001.

Gould, Stephen Jay. "The Median Isn't the Message." In *The Richness of Life: The Essential Stephen Jay Gould,* edited by Paul McGarr and Steven Rose, 26–31. New York: Norton, 2006.

Grady, Denise. "Haunted by a Gene," *New York Times,* March 10, 2020. https://www.nytimes.com/2020/03/10/health/huntingtons-disease-wexler.html.

Greco, Monica. "The Classification and Nomenclature of 'Medically Unexplained Symptoms': Conflict, Performativity and Critique." *Social Science & Medicine* 75 (2012): 2362–69. DOI: 10.1016/j.socscimed.2012.09.010.

"Guidelines for the Molecular Genetics Predictive Test in Huntington's Disease." *Journal of Medical Genetics* 31, no. 7 (1994): 555–59. DOI: 10.1136/jmg.31.7.555.

"Guidelines for the Molecular Genetics Predictive Test in Huntington's Disease." *Neurology* 44, no. 8 (1994): 1533–36.

Hache, Émilie. *Ce à quoi nous tenons*. Paris: La Découverte, 2011.

Haraway, Donna J. *The Companion Species Manifesto: Dogs, People and Significant Otherness*. Chicago: University of Chicago Press, 2003.

———. *When Species Meet*. Minneapolis: University of Minnesota Press, 2008.

Hemphill, Michael. "Pretesting for Huntington's Disease: An Overview." *Hastings Center Report* 3, no. 3 (June 1973): 12–13. DOI: 10.2307/3560596.

Hennion, Antoine, and Pierre A. Vidal-Naquet. "'Enfermer Maman!' Épreuves et arrangements: Le care comme éthique de situation." *Sciences sociales et santé* 33, no. 3 (2015): 65–90. DOI: 10.3917/sss.333.0065.

Hennion, Antoine, Pierre A. Vidal-Naquet, Franck Guichet, and Léonie Hénaut. *Une ethnographie de la relation d'aide: De la ruse à la fiction, ou comment concilier protection et autonomie*. Report for MiRe-DREES/CSI-Cerpe, 2012. http://hal-ensmp.archives-ouvertes.fr/hal-00722277.

Hermant, Émilie, and Valérie Pihet. *Le chemin des possibles. La maladie de Huntington au soin de ses usagers*. Paris: Éditions Dingdingdong, 2017.

Hölzer, Henrike. "Die Simulation von Arzt-Patienten-Kontakten in der medizinischen Ausbildung." In *Szenen des Erstkontakts zwischen Arzt und Patient*, edited by Walter Bruchhausen and Céline Kaiser, 107–17. Bonn: Bonn University Press, 2012.

Huniche, Lotte. "Moral Landscapes and Everyday Life in Families with Huntington's Disease: Aligning Ethnographic Description and Bioethics." *Social Science &*

Medicine 72, no. 11 (2011): 1810–16. DOI: 10.1016/j.socsci-med.2010.06.039.

Huntington, George. "On Chorea." *Journal of Neuropsychiatry and Clinical Neurosciences* 15, no. 1 (Winter 2003): 109–12. DOI: 10.1176/jnp.15.1.109.

Husquinet, H., G. Franck, and C. Vranckx. "Detection of Future Cases of Huntington's Chorea by the L-dopa Load Test: Experiment with Two Monozygotic Twins." *Advances in Neurology* 1 (1973): 301–10.

Jaillard, Dominique. "Plutarque et la divination: La piété d'un prêtre philosophe." *Revue de l'histoire des religions* 2 (2007): 149–69.

James, William. *The Will to Believe and Other Essays in Popular Philosophy.* New York: Dover Publications, 1956.

Jonckheere, Claude de. *83 mots pour penser l'intervention en travail social.* Geneva: Éditions IES, 2010.

Julie. *Dingdingdong,* July 9, 2013. https://dingdingdong.org/temoignages/julie/.

Kollek, Regine, and Thomas Lemke. *Der medizinische Blick in die Zukunft. Gesellschaftliche Implikationen prädiktiver Gentests.* New York: Campus Verlag, 2008.

Kristen, Maud. "Lettre de Maud Kristen au Dr Marboeuf." *Dingdingdong,* March 1, 2015. https://dingdingdong.org/departements/narration-speculative/lettre-de-maud-kristen-au-dr-marboeuf/.

Lahiri, Nayana. "The Genetic 'Gray Area' of Huntington's Disease: What Does It All Mean?" *HD Buzz,* April 22, 2011. http://en.hdbuzz.net/027.

Latour, Bruno. *On the Modern Cult of the Factish Gods.* Translated by Heather MacLean and Catherine Porter. Durham: Duke University Press, 2010.

———. *Reassembling the Social: An Introduction to Actor-Network Theory.* Oxford: Oxford University Press, 2005.

———. "Why Has Critique Run out of Steam? From Matters of Fact to Matters of Concern." *Critical Inquiry* 30, no. 2 (2004): 225–48. DOI: 10.1086/421123.

Lemke, Thomas. *Veranlagung und Verantwortung. Genetische Diagnostik zwischen Selbstbestimmung und Schicksal.* Bielefeld: Transcript Verlag, 2004.

Littré, Émile, and Charles Robin. *Dictionnaire de médicine de chirurgie, de pharmacie, de l'art vétérinaire et des sciences qui s'y rapportent.* 13th edn. Paris: J.B. Baillière et fils, 1873.

Lüdcke, Christian, and Peter Langkafel. *Breaking Bad News. Das Überbringen schlechter Nachrichten in der Medizin.* Heidelberg: Economica Verlag, 2008.

Luhmann, Niklas. Die Wissenschaft der Gesellschaft. Frankfurt am Main: Suhrkamp Verlag, 1990.

Macho, Thomas. "Was tun? Skizzen zur Wissensgeschichte der Beratung." In *Think Tanks. Die Beratung der Gesellschaft,* edited by Thomas Brandstetter, Claus Pias, and Sebastian Vehlken, 59–85. Berlin: Diaphanes, 2010.

Marks, Herbert. "Der Geist Samuels. Die biblische Kritik an prognostischer Prophetie." In *Prophetie und Prognostik,* edited by Daniel Weidner and Stefan Willer, 99–121. Berlin: Fink, 2013.

Mol, Annemarie. *The Logic of Care: Health and the Problem of Patient Choice.* London: Routledge, 2008.

Nathan, Tobie. "En psychothérapie: maladies, patients, sujets, clients ou usagers?" Paper presented at *La psychothérapie à l'épreuve de ses usagers,* Centre Devereux, Paris, France, October 12, 2006. http://www.ethnopsychiatrie.net/tobieusagers.htm.

———. *L'étranger ou le pari de l'autre.* Paris: Éditions Autrement, 2014.

———. *Psychothérapies.* Paris: Odile Jacob, 1998.

Nathan, Tobie, and Isabelle Stengers. *Doctors and Healers.* Oxford: Oxford University Press, 2018.

Novas, Carlos. *Governing "Risky" Genes: Predictive Genetics, Counselling Expertise, and the Care of the Self.* Boston Spa: British Library Document Supply Centre, 2003.

Pignarre, Philippe. *Le grand secret de l'industrie pharmaceutique*. Paris: La Découverte, 2003.

———. *Les deux médecines. Médicaments, psychotropes et suggestion thérapeutique*. Paris: La Découverte, 1995.

Pignarre, Philippe, and François Dagognet. *100 mots pour comprendre les medicaments. Comment on vous soigne*. Paris: Les Empêcheurs de penser en rond, 2005.

Pignarre, Philippe, and Isabelle Stengers. *Capitalist Sorcery: Breaking the Spell*. New York: Palgrave Macmillan, 2011.

Plutarch. *Moralia, Volume V: Isis and Osiris. The E at Delphi. The Oracles at Delphi No Longer Given in Verse. The Obsolescence of Oracles*. Translated by Frank Cole Babbitt. Cambridge: Harvard University Press, 1936.

———. *Moralia, Volume IX: Table-Talk, Books 7–9. Dialogue on Love*. Translated by Edwin L. Minar, F.H. Sandbach, and W.C. Helmbold. Cambridge: Harvard University Press, 1961.

Pollard, Jimmy. *Hurry-Up and Wait! A Cognitive Care Companion: Huntington's Disease in the Middle and more Advanced Years*. n.p.: Lulu.com, 2008.

"Recommendations for the Predictive Genetic Test in Huntington's Disease." *Clinical Genetics* 83, no. 3 (2013): 221–31. DOI: 10.1111/j.1399-0004.2012.01900.x.

Rivières, Alice. "Apeldoorn 2012." *Dingdingdong,* December 5, 2012. https://dingdingdong.org/reportages/apeldoorn-2012

Rose, Nikolas, and Carlos Novas. "Genetic Risk and the Birth of the Somatic Individual." *Economy and Society* 29, no. 4 (2000): 485–513. DOI: 10.1080/03085140050174750.

Rosenberg, Charles E. *Our Present Complaint*. Baltimore: Johns Hopkins University Press: 2007.

Sacks, Oliver. *Awakenings*. New York: Harper Perennial, 1990.

Schneider, Reto. "Wissen ist Ohnmacht." *Die Zeit,* October 12, 2000. https://www.zeit.de/2000/42/Wissen_ist_Ohnmacht.

Shelley, Mary. *Frankenstein; or, The Modern Prometheus.* Boston: Sever, Francis, & Co., 1869.

Stengers, Isabelle. *Cosmopolitics I.* Translated by Robert Bononno. Minneapolis: University of Minnesota Press, 2010.

———. *The Invention of Modern Science.* Translated by Daniel Smith. Minneapolis: University of Minnesota Press, 2000.

Tauber, Alfred I. *Patient Autonomy and the Ethics of Responsibility.* Cambridge: MIT Press, 2005.

Thomas, S. "Ethics of a Predictive Test for Huntington's Chorea." *British Medical Journal* 284, no. 6326 (May 1982): 1383–85. DOI: 10.1136/bmj.284.6326.1383.

Toulmin, Stephen. "How Medicine Saved the Life of Ethics." *Perspectives in Biology and Medicine* 25, no. 4 (1982): 736–50. DOI: 10.1353/pbm.1982.0064.

"Une politique de l'hérésie. Entretien avec Isabelle Stengers." *Vacarme* 19, no. 2 (2002): 4–13. https://vacarme.org/article263.html.

Unité Expérimentale Alice Rivières. "#1 Dr Marboeuf sur la maladie de Huntington (Huntington's disease)." *YouTube,* October 21, 2013. https://youtu.be/S1WqbR-B9a6Q.

Weil-Dubuc, Paul-Loup. "Les servitudes du droit de savoir: Autour du diagnostic présymptomatique." *La Vie des Idées,* 15 October 2013. http://www.laviedesidees.fr/les-servitudes-du-droit-de-savoir.html.

Wexler, Alice. *Mapping Fate: A Memoir of Family, Risk, and Genetic Research.* Berkeley: University of California Press, 1996.

Wexler, Nancy. "Clairvoyance and Caution: Repercussions from the Human Genome Project." In *The Code of Codes: Scientific and Social Issues in the Human Genome*

Project, edited by Daniel J. Kevles and Leroy E. Hood, 211–43. Cambridge: Harvard University Press, 1992.

———. "The Oracle of DNA." In *Molecular Genetics in Diseases of Brain, Nerve, and Muscle*, edited by L.P. Rowland, D.S. Wood, E.A. Schon, and S. DiMauro, 429–42. Oxford: Oxford University Press, 1989.

———. "The Tiresias Complex: Huntington's Disease as a Paradigm of Testing for Late-Onset Disorders." *FASEB Journal* 6, no. 10 (1992): 2820–25. DOI: 10.1096/fasebj.6.10.1386047.